Confronting AIDS through Literature

Confronting AIDS through Literature

■ The Responsibilities of Representation

EDITED BY
Judith Laurence Pastore

UNIVERSITY OF ILLINOIS PRESS
URBANA AND CHICAGO

© 1993 by the Board of Trustees of the University of Illinois
Manufactured in the United States of America
1 2 3 4 5 C P 5 4 3 2 1

This book is printed on acid-free paper.

Library of Congress Cataloging-in-Publication Data

Confronting AIDS through literature : the responsibilities of
   representation / edited by Judith Laurence Pastore.
        p. cm.
     Includes bibliographical references.
     ISBN 0-252-01989-X (cloth : alk. paper).—ISBN 0-252-06294-9
   (pbk.)
      1. American literature—20th century—History and criticism.
   2. AIDS (Disease) in literature.   3. Literature and society—United
   States—History—20th century.   4. American literature—20th
   century—Study and teaching.   5. AIDS (Disease) in literature—Study
   and teaching.   6. Gay men in literature—Study and teaching.
   7. AIDS (Disease)—Literary collections.   8. Gay men—Literary
   collections.   9. Gay men in literature.   I. Pastore, Judith
   Laurence, 1933–
   PS169.A42C66 1993
   810.9′356—dc20   92-31606
                                                               CIP

How many years have we waited for a real breakthrough, for some real shining light of hope? I've been living and breathing this subject for so long that I lose sight of just how remarkable this is. It will be possible to live with HIV infection and *not* be overwhelmed by it. It *is* possible to postpone becoming ill. And it *is* possible to live amidst this tragedy, to hold our heads high, to keep our eyes focused on the future. Though I can't know what the future may hold, I do know that for now, here, I am *well*, I am in control, and I have confidence.

Paul Reed, *The Q Journal: A Treatment Diary*

Contents

Introduction

As a culture, we have grown accustomed to privileging certain discourses over others—the words uttered by scientists and technologists are attended to with much more respect than those of artists. Yet long after many of the early scientific reports and research surrounding Acquired Immune Deficiency Syndrome (AIDS) have ceased to be important, many of the artistic works it has produced will continue to speak to us not just about this horrific modern disease but also about what it means to be human.

Although currently out of fashion, didactic literature has traditionally played a crucial role in voicing cultural values. Artistic radar picks up signals when values are being threatened or when they need to be changed to accommodate new realities. AIDS, often mislabeled a plague,[1] constitutes a new reality that challenges many existing values. Artists have responded to this challenge in every medium available. This collection brings together some of the creative writings AIDS has inspired and examines many of the problems associated with writing about such a horrific disease. Finally, it offers three essays detailing how literary AIDS can be used in the classroom.

Because many persons with AIDS (PWAs) in America were at first socially marginalized gay men, drug users, or Haitians, literary AIDS had to contend with enormous prejudice in the hegemonic culture. References to gay sexual practices aroused feelings of discomfort, if not outright disgust, in many mainstream readers. Many felt the same disgust for IV drug users, whereas Haitian PWAs were victimized by America's endemic racism. Even when middle-class heterosexuals contracted the Human Immunodeficiency Virus (HIV) through blood transfusions or through the Factor VIII hemophiliacs take, its transmission by blood or semen still placed it squarely in taboo territory for many people. This made it difficult for even well-known authors to be heard. In her short essay in this volume, "Writing about AIDS for Young Adults," M. E. Kerr, author of many best-selling adolescent novels, recounts the uncertainty she felt when in 1984 she began *Night Kites,* a novel focusing on a disease still called by some at the time GRIDS, or Gay-Related Immune Deficiency Syndrome.[2]

Apart from the sexist and racist prejudices surrounding AIDS, the disease's exceptionally grim nature makes it a topic that many people prefer to avoid thinking about altogether. Even those familiar with Aristotelian justifications for tragedy question whether anyone really wants to read creative literature about AIDS. Andrew Holleran, in *Ground Zero* (1988), was one of the first authors to confront the many problems facing those who write about AIDS, including the reluctance of many to read about such a terrible disease. He ultimately concluded that the horrors of AIDS were beyond the scope of fiction.

Sharon Mayes fell victim to this perceived readership problem. Her essay in this collection, "It Can Happen: An Essay on the Denial of AIDS," voices her anger and dismay over the rejection of her story which appears in part 2, "The Federal Bureau of Blood Inspection," by a publisher who had requested "something" on AIDS but told her that what she had written was "too depressing." Many people have reacted the same way when they learned about this collection: "Who wants to read about such a horrible disease?" "Doesn't the media assault us enough every day with worldwide tragedy without your asking us to share the suffering of PWAs and their loved ones?" Many people question whether reading imaginative literature about AIDS will really create more compassion and understanding. And perhaps more crucially, they question whether reading such literature will lead to active attempts to combat the disease.

If Aristotle was correct, then the artistic representation of human suffering shouldn't make us depressed. Rather, it is the avoidance of genuine tragedy and the substitution of glib sentimentality that diminishes us. Literature about AIDS does not make us feel better because someone else is in pain; rather, the imaginative depiction of other people exhibiting a nobility of spirit makes us proud to be human and willing to imitate their endurance and strength of character. Tragedy also reminds us of our frail mortality when it dramatizes instances of weakness and evil.

Our century has produced technologies capable of destroying life as we know it. It has also witnessed the Holocaust. Now we are faced with AIDS, which threatens to endure long into the twenty-first century and whose conquest requires the best instincts of people everywhere. Nothing in recent history has so challenged our reliance on modern science nor emphasized our vulnerability before nature. People have always turned to the imagination to deal with the seemingly mysterious forces of nature, and AIDS has been no exception. Too often the fearful imaginings prompted by this new epidemic have led to evil and violence against PWAs and those who are HIV-positive. One of the earliest tasks literary AIDS took on was combating the multiple untruths and prejudices surrounding the disease. From the beginning then, literary AIDS has had many educational goals: to preach the need for safe sex and clean needles, to dispel unwarranted fears, and to win sympathy for the infected and their loved ones.

In spite of early indifference and the many difficulties associated with representing the realities of this new disease, in little over a decade an impressive number of works in a variety of genres has emerged. Early on, gay artists began trying to educate about the need for safe sex. By March 1983, when AIDS was already well entrenched in New York, Larry Kramer's fiery essay "1,112 and Counting" lashed out at the indifference of the government, the media, and the gay community itself, warning: "If we don't act immediately, then we face our approaching doom" (50). His newspaper essay, published in the gay journal *New York Native,* was reprinted around the country and had great impact on AIDS policy, particularly in San Francisco (Shilts 245). Kramer's play *The Normal Heart* (1985) was one of the earliest to dramatize AIDS, as was William Hoffman's *As Is* (1985). In *The Normal Heart* Kramer dramatizes the founding of the Gay Men's Health Crisis (GMHC), a volunteer New York organization devoted to helping PWAs in numerous ways. Throughout, Kramer lashes out at government inaction at all levels which made gay self-help groups so crucial.

In many instances, literary AIDS has sought to combat the scapegoating of PWAs. Two early AIDS novels, for example, Toby Johnson's *Plague* (1987) and Jed Bryan's *Cry in the Desert* (1987), depict plots of deliberate genocide against gay PWAs, in the hope of preventing persecution. Nevertheless, around the country violence against gays is on the rise. Nationally, according to the Washington-based National Gay and Lesbian Task Force, 7,031 antigay incidents were reported in 1989, with 1,329 taking place on campuses and 1,078 directed against PWAs. Between January 1 and August 1, 1990, the Fenway Community Health Center's Victim Recovery Program recorded 50 hate crimes against gays in Boston alone, up from 17 the previous year (Longcope, "Reports" 1). And in 1992, when 25 members of the Irish-American Gay, Lesbian, and Bisexual Committee tried to walk in South Boston's annual St. Patrick's Day parade, they ran a gauntlet of obscenities, threats, and insults from many of the 600,000 spectators.

In a June 1991 report by the American Civil Liberties Union, Nan D. Hunter, its principal author, expressed surprise that even people aware that AIDS is not spread casually still have prevented PWAs from holding jobs or getting housing, insurance, and medical care. In fact, 30 percent of the reported cases of discrimination were not against PWAs themselves, but against those who took care of them or were otherwise considered at risk. "The stigma has a life of its own," Hunter believes. "It is irrational. Discrimination not only persists, but increases—people's behavior has not changed even though their knowledge has" (qtd. in Hilts).

Can literary AIDS overcome the homophobia and racism which often underlie attitudes toward PWAs? In a report released on August 21, 1990, to President Bush and congressional leaders, the fifteen-member National Commission on AIDS found severe hardship for PWAs in much of rural America. Several members had studied rural areas in Texas and Georgia and found that AIDS education in those areas is "virtually nonexistent and desperately needed." Because people there do not understand the disease, they repeatedly violate the human rights of those infected, who are often rejected by their employers, their friends, their family and their church (*Boston Globe* 22 Aug. 1990: 24). Even when many people learn the truth about how AIDS is spread, their strong homophobic or racist convictions make them blame the "victims." Pat Buchanan, in Georgia for the 1992 presidential primary, reiterated his earlier claim that AIDS was "nature's form of retribution" against homosexuals (*Boston Globe* 28 Feb. 1992: 12). Many artists share the fervent hope that what they create can combat such inhumane vilification; that their depictions of human suffering, sacrifices, and dignity will generate enough compassion to open minds and hearts previously closed to pleas that all America unite to combat AIDS.

Susan Sontag, in *AIDS and Its Metaphors* (1989), points to another dangerous untruth about AIDS—the conviction many share that, like the plague and tuberculosis, AIDS is a highly contagious disease which can be contracted from the most casual contact, such as coughing or sneezing. This erroneous assumption has created enormous physical, economic, and psychological hardships for PWAs and their families and is one of the major false beliefs literary AIDS has tried to correct. One of the best early autobiographies that dispells some of these mistaken beliefs is Barbara Peabody's *The Screaming Room* (1986), which recounts her son's illness and death. When I have assigned the book in college courses focusing on technology and values, students have said that they hated its details, but came to feel much more sympathy for PWAs. They also felt they had learned a great deal more about the disease and ultimately were glad they had been required to read it. Laurel Brodsley, Sandra W. Stephan, and Joseph Cady have also taught literary AIDS in various university courses, and their essays in part 3 offer many creative suggestions about how these writings can be employed in different educational settings to bring home to many more people the truths about this disease.

Dystopian visions have traditionally been used to identify and combat dangerous social trends, and a number of early AIDS works are in this mode.[3] The horrific experiences that one heterosexual couple endure in Sharon Mayes's "Federal Bureau of Blood Inspection" portend a dystopian nightmare in which those with HIV suffer total loss of freedom. Jed A. Bryan's essay in this volume, "Crying 'Wolf!': The Genesis of an AIDS Disaster Epic," explains why his early AIDS novel *A Cry in the Desert* (1987) presents a similar nightmare vision of a world where genocide is deliberately used against gays. In real life, homophobic youths in a Las Vegas parking lot began taunting the lover of one of Bryan's friends, calling him "faggot" and "death spreader." They then deliberately ran over him with a car and killed him.

Beyond its didactic goals, does literary AIDS have other, more traditional literary aims? As an expressive medium, it most certainly does, as countless artists have used it to assuage their grief and to bear witness to those destroyed. Paul Monette, in his memoir *Borrowed Time* (1988) and his poems *Love Alone: 18 Elegies for Rog* (1988), typifies those who have turned to literature to memorialize a lost loved one. "The Very Same," reprinted in part 2 from *Love Alone,* furiously rejects the suggestion that it is *"time to turn the page."* In his preface to *Love Alone,* Monette insists: "I would rather have this volume filed under AIDS than under Poetry, because if these words speak to anyone they are for those who are mad with loss, to let them know they are not alone."

Like Monette, many writers have turned to poetry to express grief, outrage, despair, love, and hope. In this collection, the African-American author Melvin Dixon uses the viewpoint of an elderly woman in "Aunt Ida Pieces a Quilt" to connect the death of Junie, with his "too-tight dungarees, his blue choir robe," with the 14,000 dead persons memorialized in the NAMES Project Quilt. In his prose-poem "Voices," Jed A. Bryan experiments with echoes of the clichés and prejudices surrounding the disease, hoping that his contrapuntal texture will make us rehear with greater sympathy the everyday language of AIDS. William Greenway's "Epidemic" compares in startling imagery nature's healthy growth cycles with the malignant cycles of HIV. And the eminent novelist and poet May Sarton, who responded immediately to a request for submissions to this collection, urges that everyone else respond immediately with the best response to AIDS: "Love. Love. Love. Love."

As with all expressive literature, artistic worth varies enormously. In "What are the Responsibilities of Representing AIDS?" I discuss some of the problems associated with writing and judging literature about AIDS. One aim of this collection is to show that, in spite of the short time people have been aware of the disease, much variety and breadth already exists in literature of this kind. In this regard, the number of selections here by women show that literary AIDS has not just been the purview of gay men. Accounts by mothers who had lost sons were among the first forms of writing to appear. The earliest novel about AIDS, Dorothy Bryant's *A Day in San Francisco* (1983), voices a mother's fear that some terrible new illness threatens her gay son. Soon wives were writing about husbands. Elizabeth Fox, in *Thanksgiving, An AIDS Journal* (1990), writes about her bisexual husband's death from AIDS and her struggle with mixed feelings of rage, compassion, and fear that her son would be stigmatized if anyone were to find out. More recently, women have begun writing about their own infection. Elizabeth Glaser, who made a stirring speech at the 1992 Democratic National Convention, and whose husband Paul Michael Glaser starred in the television series "Starsky and Hutch," got transfusion AIDS while delivering her first child. Her account *In the Absence of Angels* (1991) documents how even those seemingly protected by fame and fortune can be ostracized once people learn they carry HIV.

San Francisco's "Atomic Comic" Fran Peavey, known for her activist politics, also wrote about her own infection and how few facilities at the time were equipped to deal with female AIDS patients. In her four-year journal *A Shallow Pool of Time* (1989), Peavey describes how, like many women early on, she was convinced that she was "gender-immune": "one gets it from bathhouses where gay men do things that I cannot imagine" (1). Her view changed when she contracted transfusion AIDS, thereby challenging her prior commitment to non-violence. "What will it take to wake this country—this world—up?" she asks (51). "Where is the national will to discuss, to educate, to heal and care?" (52). According to the World Health Organization, approximately 3 million women and children around the world will die of AIDS in the 1990s. In the United States, AIDS in women has been steadily increasing, becoming the fifth-leading cause of death in women of child-bearing years. In New York and New Jersey, AIDS is already the leading cause of death among women 15 to 34 (Longcope, "AIDS" 36). This strongly suggests that coping with the risks of the epidemic will become a staple in any work relating to women's lives. Elizabeth Gershman of Knights Press, when I spoke with her on the phone about this collection, said she believes that it is impossible to write any kind of realistic fiction today without including AIDS. And one finds fear of contracting it does at least get mentioned in most contemporary realistic fiction. Joel Redon's novel *Bloodstream* (1989) depicts without sentimentality a young man with HIV who returns home to make peace with the demons of his youth. Chapter 11, reprinted here, depicts a feverish bout in which twenty-five-year-old Peter relives scenes of childhood guilt, accompanied by a nagging litany of present guilt.

In a totally different vein, Larry Ebmeier and David B. Feinberg use their talent for humor to represent other realities of the AIDS experience. Ebmeier's novel *Tweeds* (1987), published under the pseudonym Clayton R. Graham, is a gay bildungsroman in which a shy, pudgy, midwestern farmboy grows up loving his handsome best friend. They are reunited years later in Chicago, but by then the friend has AIDS. Ebmeier introduces us in "Requiem Evita" to the quotidian details of gay life—the warmth of friendship, the delight in wit, the relish of the absurd, the youthful joys that AIDS cuts short as one friend after another becomes affected. Replacing anger or horror with quiet humor, he invites us to share his personal responses. David B. Feinberg's satiric humor is very different. Whereas Ebmeier's style reflects the gentler world of his rural Nebraskan youth, Feinberg's echoes the neurotic absurdities of today's urban existence. Author of the highly acclaimed, darkly comic *Eighty-sixed* (1989), a before-and-after AIDS novel, Feinberg continues, in the story reprinted here, "Despair," his dramatization of the experiences of gay, young Manhattanite B.J. Rosenthal. This time Rosenthal faces with typical grim humor his acute anxiety about getting the HIV antibody test.

The poet Michael Lynch, who died of AIDS in July 1991, employs a highly imaginative approach to writing about the disease. Writing in the third person, he critiques his own AIDS poem "The Terror of Resurrection." Because he became too ill to deliver this critique himself, it was delivered for him at the 1988 meeting of the Modern Language Association by the eminent literary critic Eve Kosofsky Sedgwick.

In a look at how much gay relationships do and do not resemble traditional marriages, British author David Rees's story "Spring and

Fall" dramatizes the strong bonds between an older PWA and his young lover, who struggles with the temptation of sexual betrayal. Rees's story also presents an unsentimental glimpse of daily life for a PWA and his loved one which is not depressing: a friend drops in for drinks, and funny stories about shared memories are recalled.

This picture of a PWA coping with humor and dignity is fairly typical. Contrary to what many people might imagine, literary AIDS is not a monotonous record of human misery and passive victimization. Indeed, many of the writers represented in this collection have used their creative abilities to dramatize a variety of survival strategies. David Feinberg's *Spontaneous Combustion* (1991), in which "Despair" appears, presents sketch after sketch showing how B.J. copes with being HIV-positive, while Paul Reed's *Q Journal* (1991) details his treatment with the banned Compound Q. Although he experiences a variety of physical and psychological problems, Reed's attitude most of the time is optimistic. When I have assigned this book to college students, they have been amazed that a book about HIV infection and treatment was not altogether depressing. As more drugs and alternative therapies become available, it is to be hoped that this aspect of literary AIDS will become even more prominent and will provide valuable support to PWAs and their loved ones.

Another way literary AIDS has provided enormous support has been its record of the quest for spiritual solace by those whom modern science could not heal. In *And the Band Played On* (1987), Randy Shilts documents the pilgrimage San Francisco native and PWA Bill Kraus makes to Lourdes after other "miracle" cures fail. A lapsed Catholic, Bill felt it wasn't cool to believe in faith healing, but still he hoped for a miracle:

> Bill stared toward the Virgin, and he began to see her as the archetypal mother, not the literal mother of God, but the source of all nourishment and hope. He could speak to that mother, and it would mean something. At last, he could pray, and the words would not be empty.
>
> He realized that the bitterness he had held against the church had alienated him from this elemental source of strength. He had been separated from the font of love and forgiveness that Jesus had to offer, and it was not right. God knew that. It all was very clear to Bill now, and for the first time in many years he prayed. (538)

Toby Johnson's essay in this collection shares this aspect of literary AIDS. His *Plague: A Novel About Healing* (1987) presents a dystopic vision of homophobic persecution, but in "Facing the Edge: AIDS as a Source of Spiritual Wisdom," he grapples instead with the longing many gays feel for spiritual answers.

One of the earliest to write a novel focusing on AIDS—*Facing It* (1984)—Paul Reed wonders in his short essay "Early AIDS Fiction" why so few other novelists followed suit.[4] Don Shewey, who has edited anthologies of gay dramas, points out how, in contrast, "drama has taken the lead in educating audiences and showing concern for the afflicted" (5). In 1990, the Theatre Communications Group, the national organization for nonprofit theatre, published a number of these AIDS plays in an anthology *The Way We Live Now*. Michael Cunningham notes the vast change in how theater treats gay issues since he saw *The Boys in the Band* in 1970: "AIDS has slammed in a new perspective. These days, most theater by or about gay people is fueled by a sorrow so intricately threaded with rage that the two emotions have started to feel like the same thing" (1).

There are several reasons why theater took the lead, besides the obvious fact that plays usually can be written more quickly than novels. Many persons involved with theater have had friends die of AIDS. Original plays tend to be produced first in large cities which usually have a sizeable gay population. Finally, the conventional novel, with its middle-class orientation and need for closure, in many ways distorts the AIDS experience. Tragedy and comedy, with their accepted exaggerations—their ability to put the horrors of the present in a more timeless perspective—are perhaps better suited to depict the disease. In this sense, Randy Shilts's *And the Band Played On* is so compelling because it combines new journalism techniques with the bitter irony of formal tragedy. Like watching Oedipus, we cannot escape the knowledge eluding the characters, which makes all they say and do reverberate with ominous prescience.

On the other hand, not all the news from the theater has been good. Commenting on AIDS dramas generally, the *Boston Globe* theater critic Kevin Kelly believes that some plays have tended to exploit the disease as a way of simply adding trendiness to their productions. He cites Wendy Wasserstein's *Heidi Chronicles*, in which Peter Patrone's grief for a lover dying of AIDS is, according to Kelly, used merely to create intimacy between Patrone and Heidi (39–40). In contrast, Peter Barnes's *Red Noses*, although set in the plague years of the fourteenth century, has prompted some people, including Sam Coale, who writes about the play in this collection, to see it as a cautionary AIDS allegory. James W. Jones, though, in his essay "The Sick Homosexual: AIDS and Gays on the American Stage and Screen" included here, finds few sincere attempts early on to represent the realities of AIDS in theater, television, or cinema. Still, as the bibliography shows, television has gradually begun to offer more dramatizations of the disease. Whereas Ron Cowen and Daniel Lipman's "Early Frost" (1985) was considered a radical departure for commercial television, a number of shows in 1992 focused on AIDS. ABC's "Life Goes On," for example, introduced Jesse, an HIV-positive character (ten out of twenty-two episodes on the show deal with HIV in one way or another). In one episode, Jesse goes to an AIDS hospice where one of the residents is played by Michael Kearns, who is himself HIV-positive. In addition, two episodes of NBC's "Sisters" focus on an HIV-positive teacher whom some parents want fired. Hollywood, on the other hand, keeps promising to take the disease more seriously, but with the epidemic already in its second decade, only one commercial AIDS film, *Longtime Companion,* has been made.[5] Hollywood's refusal to offer more representations of the disease's realities are prompting mounting anger from AIDS activists.

This resistance by those in power in Hollywood to make major films about AIDS brings us back to the initial problem of asking literature to confront such a grim disease. Michael Denneny, in "AIDS Writing and the Creation of a Gay Culture," included here, can find no parallel to literary AIDS. Writing about the Holocaust has often come to light only long after the event, whereas literary AIDS is about the now: "it is reports from the combat zone." Comparing AIDS writing to *The Diary of Anne Frank,* Denneny states that Anne did not know what would happen, and we who read about it cannot change what did. But those who write about AIDS know what is happening and want desperately to change it.

The selections in this volume represent the different ways people have used literature to confront the realities of AIDS. Some use traditional literary genres, some are experimental. Others demonstrate how this literature can be used in a variety of educational settings. Still others explore many of the problematic issues connected to literature about the disease. How should such writings be judged? How explicit should their descriptions of sexual practices be? Whose perspective should take precedence and whose can be trusted to represent the truth? And finally, will the literary genres represented and discussed here be the best imaginative tools in the future for reaching young persons at risk, particularly those of color, or will other entertainment modes be more effective?

Unless persons of good will unite to effect genuine healing, the metaphors of AIDS will become a reality as the many illnesses in our culture are left to fester and infect our national spirit. Nothing can be done as long as one group is set against another—straights against gays, whites against blacks, men against women. If literary AIDS can contribute in a small way to bringing together in understanding those who are now divided by either ignorance or bigotry, then the efforts of all the contributors to this volume will have been worthwhile.

All profits over publishing costs will go to the National Association of People with AIDS (NAPWA), 1412 K Street, N.W., Washington, D.C. 20005, which provides information about treatment, social service, financial, and legal options; training and technical assistance to local AIDS service organizations; and national and local advocacy for people with HIV disease.

Notes

1. Laurel Brodsley, in "Teaching about AIDS and Plagues: A Reading List from the Humanities," describes her course on the literature of plagues and AIDS, one of whose aims is to show students the differences between the two phenomena.

2. The Centers for Disease Control (CDC) substituted AIDS for GRIDS in 1982 "because people other than homosexual men also began to develop the condition" (Connor and Kingman 14).

3. For an analysis of early AIDS literature, see Shaun O'Connor's "The Big One: Literature Discovers AIDS."

4. Few novels besides Bryant's *A Day in San Francisco* (1983), Reed's *Facing It* (1984), and Reed's safe-sex erotica under the pseudonym Max Exander *SafeStud* (1985) and *LoveSex* (1986) appeared before 1987. From that time, many have begun to appear. See the annotated bibliography for a partial list.

5. Richard Natale, writing in the *Village Voice*, believes the reason Hollywood is avoiding AIDS is that "Movies generally deal in closure and resolution. AIDS has thus far resisted making itself accessible in that way" (70). He then discusses a number of AIDS film projects. Judith Guest (*Ordinary People*) is supposedly writing something for Disney, and Brian Hohlfeld is working on *Just People* for Columbia, about a doctor who falls in love with a woman with AIDS. At Warner, William Hoffman, author of the play *As Is*, is doing a script for Whoopi Goldberg about a black woman with AIDS. Joel Schumacher's script *Intimate Relations*, about a young man confronting his family with both his gayness and AIDS, however, went from studio to studio until Paramount finally agreed to do it, but only as a small film. Schumacher objected, "because a 'small' film would only have been seen by an audience that already knows about AIDS. I wanted to reach a wider audience" (qtd. in Natale 70). Alice Hoffman's novel *At Risk* was optioned by producer Lawrence Gordon, but the option was allowed to expire. Barbra Streisand wanted to produce, direct and co-star as the Mathilde Krim–like doctor in Larry Kramer's play *The Normal Heart*, but contractual disagreements between her and Kramer have reportedly put the project on hold. Randy Shilts's *And the*

Band Played On has been picked up by HBO, but the script originally commissioned by NBC, which they found "too gay," is being totally rewritten, so it won't be shown for at least another year. Shilts's work was first strongly considered by Twentieth Century Fox before they pulled out at the last minute. As Paula Treichler pointed out in her comments on this text: "Hollywood films that appear to deal with AIDS" do so in a "displaced way." For example, AIDS will get mentioned in reviews of *Aliens, The Fly,* and *Fatal Attraction,* but not as a subject of its own.

Works Cited

The annotated bibliography contains information about the specific works on literary AIDS mentioned in the Introduction.

Connor, Steve, and Sharon Kingman. *In Search for the Virus,* rev. ed. New York: Penguin, 1989.

Cunningham, Michael. "After AIDS, Gay Art Aims for a New Reality." *New York Times* 26 Apr. 1992, sec. 2: 1.

Hilts, Philip J. "AIDS Bias Grows Faster Than Disease, Study Says." *New York Times* 17 June 1990: A20.

Kelly, Kevin. "AIDS treated too often as a subplot." *The Boston Globe* 16 Apr. 1989: B39–40.

Kramer, Larry. "1,112 and Counting." *Reports from the Holocaust.* New York: St. Martin's Press, 1989. 33–51.

Longcope, Kay. "AIDS threat to women increasing." *The Boston Globe* 23 Aug. 1990: 33.

———. "Reports of antigay violence rising in state, nation." *The Boston Globe* 7 June 1990: 19.

Natale, Richard. "And the Cameras Rolled On. Why You Are Not Seeing Movies About AIDS." *The Village Voice* 20 Feb. 1990: 67.

O'Connor, Shaun. "The Big One: Literature Discovers AIDS." *The AIDS Epidemic: Private Rights and the Public Interest.* Ed. Padraig O'Malley. Boston: Beacon Press, 1989. 485–506.

Peavey, Fran. *A Shallow Pool of Time: An HIV+ Woman Grapples with the AIDS Epidemic.* San Francisco: New Society Publishers, 1990.

Shewey, Don. "AIDS on Stage: Comfort, Sorrow, Anger." *The New York Times* 21 June 1987: H5.

Shilts, Randy. *And the Band Played On.* New York: St. Martin's Press, 1987.

Sontag, Susan. *AIDS and Its Metaphors.* New York: Farrar, Straus and Giroux, 1989.

PART ONE

Literary AIDS: What Are the Responsibilities?

■ JUDITH LAURENCE PASTORE

What Are the Responsibilities of Representing AIDS?

The AIDS epidemic has forced us to confront many weaknesses in our seemingly advanced Western culture. One of them is the problematic role of the modern artist as both prophet and pariah. Another is the assumption by many that most artists are gay or lesbian. Many people have heard the contention that Hemingway wrote his macho texts to prove that, though an artist, he was still a "real man." For many authors, to write about AIDS is to risk confirming this majority prejudice. Still, it is very difficult to be an artist today and ignore the disease. Many artists have contracted HIV or have already died. "Three lives in arts, three lives cut short," a headline in the December 1, 1989, *Boston Globe* proclaims, and almost daily one reads about memorials to dead novelists, poets, songwriters, photographers, choreographers, designers, playwrights. As of November 1989, Key West, Florida, one-time home to Ernest Hemingway and Tennessee Williams, had a higher percentage of AIDS cases among its population of 27,000 than San Francisco, New York, and Miami (*Vero Beach Press Journal* 5 Nov. 1989: 1). Indeed, insurance companies consider artists one of the high-risk groups for AIDS. Blue Cross/Blue Shield, for example, raised the rates for the Boston-based Massachusetts Cultural Alliance by 70 percent two years in a row. Over thirty different companies told the Alliance's agent that "artists are a particularly difficult group to insure," with half of the insurers mentioning AIDS as the reason (Grant 74).

Because of the popular association of AIDS with artists, even involving oneself with an AIDS project presents some risks. The lesbian novelist Sarah Schulman, whose *People in Trouble* (1990) depicts a love triangle against the background of AIDS, relates that most straight artists she knows are reluctant to get involved in AIDS activism.

When I came to ACT UP I came to it as an artist, wanting to bring the arts community which was being affected by AIDS into activism, and I found that the only way that people would do that was to perform their work at a benefit, or mention AIDS in their work. And that was very few people, that was only gay people. But straight artists refused to walk into a room of 500 homosexuals, or stand on the picket line with them. (Loewenstein 22)

In *People in Trouble,* she imagines a radical group called "Justice," modeled four years ago on the way she wanted ACT UP to be:

However, in the interim ACT UP has outwitted me, and become more than even I imagined. So for example, in the book I imagined these 40 timid men nervously disrupting a service in St. Patrick's Cathedral. Well, the reality was, right before the book came out, ACT UP had this huge demonstration of 7000 angry people at St. Patrick's Cathedral. (Loewenstein 22)

The late James Baldwin was asked about using art to educate. Questioned if he would ever stop writing novels with a message, he replied: "You take risks you don't ordinarily take" ("James Baldwin"). When I was an English major in the fifties the fashionable attitude was the modernist conviction that art should be "above" politics. As students we soon understood that we were supposed to look down on "message" literature such as *Uncle Tom's Cabin* or *The Jungle.* Great art was its own justification. The priests—there were few priestesses in those days—of high art like Joyce's Stephen Dedalus deliberately sought to remain aloof.

Literary AIDS, on the other hand, reinforces the postmodernist conviction that just as there can be no separation between private and public, so also there can be no separation between art and politics. The recent battles in museums concerning certain exhibitions and between some members of Congress and the embattled National Endowment for the Arts bear this out. Schulman insists that a "major theme in *People in Trouble* is that it is impossible to write a gay book without discussing AIDS in some depth" (Loewenstein 22). Christopher Bram, whose *In Memory of Angel Clare* (1989) recounts grief for a lover lost to AIDS, also believes any contemporary novel has to "have some acknowledgment of it": "It would be interesting to see a novel where AIDS is present, but not in the foreground. In Gary Indiana's new novel, *Horse Crazy,* AIDS is just in the background; it's a very thick background. I think there will be more of that" (Gambone 16).

The process that novelist David Leavitt describes in his article "The Way I Live Now" epitomizes the struggle some gay writers have gone through to overcome their reluctance to write about AIDS. Leavitt's novel *The Lost Language of Cranes* (1986) deals openly with gay anxiety in a heterosexual culture. But when it came to AIDS, Leavitt did not want to read or write fiction about it. At first he resented people asking why he had not written about AIDS, explaining: "Because I had published a book of short stories and a novel that dealt with the themes of homosexuality and illness, I suppose they assumed the subject would come naturally to me. So what? I'd shout back. I'm not obligated to write about *anything*. Only if and when I was inspired to write about AIDS would I write about it" ("The Way I Live Now" 30). Leavitt changed his mind when he read Susan Sontag's story "The Way We Live Now" (1986). "Up to that point, reading fiction about AIDS had seemed to me akin to being shown a brick wall somewhere in the distance and then, at full speed, being hurled into it" ("The Way I Live Now" 30).

Sontag's story, told from a multiple perspective by the friends of a man dying of AIDS, goes beyond horror and grief to the way people cope with the disease. Leavitt describes the story's effect on him: "its long sentences swirled madly around the never-named disease, just as the characters—dozens of them—swirled around their suffering friend, arguing, comforting, annoying each other, giving each other their anxieties, their metaphors, their lies" ("The Way I Live Now" 30). "The Way We Live Now" offered Leavitt the possibility of catharsis. By lifting AIDS out of the realm of sex and relating it to the larger human context of death itself, whose chain of existence is inexorably linked to human sexuality, Sontag attempted to combat the moral onus afflicting AIDS.

In contrast to his reaction to Sontag's story, Leavitt was appalled by the work of writers such as William F. Buckley, who once suggested that HIV-positive persons should have their buttocks and forearms branded with a "scarlet A" (A27), or Christopher Lehmann-Haupt who, when reviewing Sontag's *AIDS and Its Metaphors* for the *New York Times,* insisted that people should really respond by changing their sexual behavior to more "conventional forms" (Leavitt, "The Way I Live Now" 31). Discovering that the language surrounding AIDS frequently stigmatizes its carriers, Leavitt finally decided to respond, and AIDS is prominent in many of the stories in his collection *A Place I've Never Been* (1990).

Leavitt's decision to respond to AIDS prejudice through art characterizes many current projects, some of which have been involved in heated controversy. This controversy raises another question surrounding the use of art to educate about AIDS: must literary AIDS conform to outside needs because of the emergency? Should the government oversee what is produced in the interest of the "common good"? The former Soviet Union, after the 1917 revolution, preached a doctrine of common good, and we know what happened to its literary output. Awareness of this danger is what makes crucial the outcome of the current controversy over the role of government funding for art.

Early in the epidemic, controversy focused mainly on more direct aspects of AIDS education—government pamphlets explaining the need for safe sex, condom use, and clean needles. Since 1989, however, attempts to heighten public awareness through visual art have aroused heated debates: for example, the uproar over Andres Serrano's "Piss Christ," a photograph of a crucifix immersed in a jar of the artist's urine, which appeared in a show funded by the NEA early in 1989, at the Southeastern Center for Contemporary Arts in North Carolina. Provoked, Senator Jesse Helms of North Carolina and Representative William E. Dannemeyer of California spearheaded federal initiatives against public "depictions of sadomasochism, homo-eroticism, the sexual exploitation of children or individuals engaged in sex acts, and which, when taken as a whole do not have serious literary, artistic, political, or scientific merit" (qtd. in Leavitt, "Fears" 27). For a time, all recipients of NEA grants had to agree in writing that their works would conform to these federal guidelines. A second outburst arose when the Corcoran Gallery in Washington, D.C., cancelled an exhibit of photographs with explicit homoerotic content by the late Robert Mapplethorpe—an exhibit that has created controversy wherever it has been shown.

Another controversy involved a $10,000 grant the NEA gave to Artists Space, a private, non-profit arts institution in Manhattan, to put on an AIDS show called "Witnesses: Against Our Vanishing," which opened on November 16, 1989. When John E. Frohnmayer, then NEA chairman, was informed of the show's content, he decided that it violated the federal prohibition. After Leonard Bernstein refused to accept the National Medal of Arts in protest, Frohnmayer reversed his decision, saying the grant was for the show and not its thirty-two-page catalog, which contained five essays, one of which was David Wojnarowicz's "Post Cards from America: X–Rays from Hell." Besides fiercely attacking New York's Cardinal O'Connor, Wojnarowicz also strongly criticized Helms and Dannemeyer. Throughout the publicity surrounding the incident, Frohnmayer kept throwing out the word "political" and then taking it back, saying finally, in one of his most confusing statements, that: "If you came to us and said, 'I want to create a political polemic,' we would not fund that. If you on the other hand said, 'I want to paint a *Guernica,'* we would fund that" (*Boston Globe* 17 Nov. 1989: 91). Of course, *Guernica* happens to be both political polemic and great art.

In May 1990, the New School for Social Research in New York City sued the NEA for making grant recipients sign what came to be known as the "artistic loyalty oath." Six recipients of 1990 grants refused to sign, thereby forfeiting grants, with a dozen more signing under protest. NEA's presidentially appointed advisory board voted 17-2 on August 3, 1990, to get rid of the antiobscenity pledge, but Frohnmayer insisted that recipients, whether they signed an oath or not, had to comply with the antiobscenity law. Otherwise, he said, "the signal might be that the endowment is thumbing its nose at the law" (*Boston Globe* 4 Aug. 1990: 16). The clause has since been dropped, but in February 1992, Frohnmayer, despite all his efforts to appease conservative critics of the NEA, was forced to resign when presidential candidate Patrick Buchanan took aim at NEA expenditures.

Leavitt worries that this current attempt to "Disneyfy" art parallels Hitler's attack on "degenerate artists." He says: "The real target behind attacks on the National Endowment is not obscenity but dread of the nameless 'other' " ("Fears" 1). "Fear of change, fear of difference, fear of cultural erosion: all these fears of the extreme right mask, in fact, a deeper fear, a fear of the underground sexual desires every individual harbors (look at Jimmy Swaggart!) and for which homosexuals have traditionally been made into a catch-all symbol" ("Fears" 27).

Linda Singer's "Bodies—Pleasures—Powers" suggests one reason why it has been difficult for liberals to develop a coherent AIDS philosophy while the extreme right has continually used AIDS to berate contemporary morality. Epidemics by their very nature require that normal freedoms be sacrificed for the good of the majority—a commonsense position that is particularly hard to refute in times of emergency but is not in accordance with the traditional liberal defense of privacy and individual freedom (Singer 50–51). Can we then ask that literary AIDS simultaneously defend the rights of marginalized persons with AIDS (PWAs) and also educate the general public about the nature of the epidemic? Moreover, if some artists, in their anger at middle-class neglect and their desire to shatter complacent indifference to the disease, seek primarily to *épater les bourgeois,* won't such art only further alienate the dominant society and make it even harder to elicit sympathy for PWAs?

As the 1990s began, a renewed spirit of censorship rapidly gained ground. Underlying Helms's antiobscenity crusade is the current national debate over what are perceived as threatened family values. David Rees's short story "Spring and Fall" dramatizes the strong bonds between an older PWA and his young lover. Paul Monette depicts similar bonds in his novel *Afterlife* (1990) about three AIDS "widows." His more recent novel *Halfway Home* (1991) vividly depicts the growing love a young man with AIDS feels for another man. Both novels contain beautifully written scenes of gay sex. Even if all prejudice against gays and PWAs were removed, can heterosexuals be expected to identify sufficiently with the Other to enjoy the sensual eroticism of such moments? As with the poetry of Sappho, I believe the work's appeal depends on its imaginative power. After all, women have responded in one way or another to accounts of military exploits that they have never experienced. Moreover, whether one can enjoy homoerotic literature is one question; whether it should be censored is another.

Besides the problems of whether homoerotic content is acceptable or not, and how much literature must conform to majority values, another question is whether we judge literary AIDS by different standards because the emergency is so great. Jan Zita Grover grapples with this question in her review of Ines Rieder and Patricia Ruppelt's anthology *AIDS: The Women,* one example of the growing body of "witness" literature. After criticizing Susan Sontag's *AIDS and Its Metaphors* for ignoring the many writings about AIDS in gay subculture, and praising Bateson and Goldsby's *Thinking AIDS* as the one book she would "propel into the hands of well-intentioned but ignorant citizens," Grover flatly states that she has to assess the "witness" and "testimony" literature of AIDS differently: "I come back to the terms 'witness' and 'testimony' because I find it isn't possible to assess the individual experiences voiced here in the same way that one criticizes the developed arguments of a Susan Sontag or Mary Catherine Bateson. Each of the women contributing to *AIDS: The Women* speaks from and to a very partial impression of the epidemic" (6).

Patricia Ruppelt believes that these personal accounts "yield a certain depth and honesty absent in an impersonal approach" (Rieder and Ruppelt 11). Grover worries that this "borders perilously on subjectivism," writing that "*AIDS: The Women* overlooks the vastly different historical and cultural formations that underlie the 'testimonies' on offer" (6). Here, Grover articulates the same problem tackled in much literary criticism today—how to deal with the subjective, whether obvious or subtle, inherent in all writing. Frequently the content which agrees with the critic's views is called honesty, whereas what conflicts is dismissed as distortion.

Writing about the current literary response to AIDS, the *New York Times* critic Michael Kimmelman alludes to the problem of judging a work written for a good cause: "This is a country that prides itself on compassion but prefers the sick to die unobtrusively" (1). Many artists have tried to arouse Americans from their passivity, but unfortunately some of these literary efforts reveal, according to Kimmelman, the limitations of art "in guiding a society's conscience": "This crisis has not always brought forth the best from artists and cultural leaders" (1). In discussing feminist literary criticism in the August 16, 1990, issue of *The New York Review of Books*, Harvard professor Helen Vendler distinguishes between thematic and aesthetic content. The former may have a lasting historical and sociological interest—*Uncle Tom's Cabin, The Jungle*—but the latter will always be judged by how well the artistic imagination "creates its own verbal universe." The fundamental structures of literature, according to Vendler, are not "documentary, thematic, or ideological." "The lifting of the documentary into the symbolic, of the thematic into the syntactic is the task of art" (25).

From another perspective, the assumptions of traditional liberal humanism presuppose that literature relates to a real world, where right and wrong exist and which writers may alter for the better if their works are good enough. For Lionel Trilling, writing in *The Liberal Imagination* (1950), the novel with its ability to reeducate the moral imagination is necessary to the preservation of freedom: "there never was a time when its particular activity was so much needed, was of so much practical, political and social use—so much so that if its impulse does not respond to the need, we shall have reason to be sad not only over a waning form of art but also over our waning freedom" (222).

Trilling wrote this at the dawn of the McCarthy era, which scapegoated hundreds of artists for their "leftist" views. The underlying philosophy, going back to Plato's eviction of poets from his Republic, is that artists can influence and perhaps alter the world "out there." But this assumption runs counter to much of today's popular literary theory. For example, Derrida, the most frequently quoted poststructuralist critic, emphasizes the logocentricism of our culture, insisting along with Wittgenstein that words create reality, not vice versa, that all language is metaphoric at some point, and that everything written contains its *différance*—its opposite which alters, if not invalidates, its stated meaning.[1] If such a situation exists in texts, how can the cultural myths and assumptions about AIDS embedded in the language be weeded out? For example, anyone who reads much about AIDS soon makes the same discovery that David Leavitt did—namely, that objectivity has been singularly lacking in all kinds of writing about this disease, including supposedly objective scientific discourse. Paula Treichler, in "AIDS, Homophobia and Biomedical Discourse," details the middle-class, heterosexual, male bias in so-called scientific facts about AIDS. We are told, for example, by John Langone in a 1985 *Discover* article that "AIDS is likely to remain a gay disease" because the "rugged vagina is designed to withstand the trauma of intercourse," whereas the "vulnerable rectum" and "fragile urethra" make anal intercourse, "second only to oral sex in frequency among homosexuals," "the commonest cause of AIDS" (40–41).[2]

From a deconstructionist viewpoint, writings about AIDS always respond to other writings about AIDS: Leavitt is responding not only to Sontag, but to Buckley, Lehmann-Haupt, Langone, and all those who write or speak about AIDS. As Sarah Schulman explains, each "of the books that I've written has been a response to the other gay literature of its time" (Loewenstein 22).

Deconstruction has made us more aware of language's metaphoric distortions, and those who work in literary AIDS are especially aware of the need to eliminate negative imagery. This is what Schulman realized when she began *People in Trouble:* "The first thing that I did was to go back to fiction that had been written about large disasters, like Holocaust fiction, Hiroshima, the plague; and what I found out is that very, very little fiction was written about those events at the time they happened or even within the next forty years or so after them" (Loewenstein 23). Like Sontag, Schulman realized that using the vocabulary of other disasters betrayed the reality of the AIDS epidemic. Because AIDS is so different—because mass death is being described in the midst of the epidemic—writers are having to find new words and new ways to respond. Schulman made lists of all the aspects of the disease she knew of and then picked fifty of them for her novel: "There were things like watch alarms going off in public places so that people could take their AZT. . . . Then there are also terms that I had to decide not to use, because there's a lot of language around AIDS that's very distorting, like 'general population' or 'innocent victim' " (Loewenstein 23). Another word Schulman rejected was "Holocaust." Like many other artists, she found that conventional literary modes and genres had to be expanded to cope with the enormity of this event. Writings about prior disasters were mostly survivor memoirs and journalism. "I think that a lot of the reason is that fiction is in some ways not an appropriate form for very huge events" (Loewenstein 23). For this reason, Schulman is happy that the Houston Grand Opera has commissioned a full production of *People in Trouble* for the spring of 1993. "In a lot of ways opera is a much more appropriate form, it's so hyperbolic and huge, melodramatic" (Loewenstein 23).

Deconstructive analysis has also been helpful in showing the silences in literary AIDS: who has been left out? Whose perspective is being heard? Although many women have contributed to literary AIDS, for example, their main focus has still been gay men. And almost all contributors thus far have been middle-class whites. The preponderance of white, middle-class, gay issues central to the concerns of AIDS activists can make it difficult for other perspectives to get a fair hearing. The controversy over the third installment of the "AIDS Quarterly," broadcast on PBS on September 27, 1989, illustrates this difficulty. Furious objections by gay activists that the program showed "insensitivity to gay and minority groups" focused on two segments. One, entitled "A Question of Civil Rights," contrasted the Howard Brown Memorial Clinic in Chicago, which serves a predominantly white, middle-class, gay male clientele, with the much poorer facilities available to blacks and Hispanics. The program also showed a "shooting-gallery" for heroin addicts in the slums, where users often swap needles. The second segment, called "AIDS and the Second Sex," showed a Washington, D.C., woman named "Christie" who had contracted AIDS from her bisexual husband. Peter Jennings's concluding statement that bisexuals "don't always tell the full story to the women they're involved with" further infuriated many gays. Eric Rosenthal, political director of the Human Rights Campaign Fund, a gay lobbying group, claimed: "it says that gay men are out there spreading the disease to women—and then stealing treatment money from blacks and Hispanics. That's outrageous. It loads bullets in the gun for anyone who's inclined toward homophobia in the first place" (qtd. in Kahn 66). Jennings, a white male, did not garner as much criticism, however, as the show's female director, Renata Simone. The writer and AIDS activist Warren Blumenfeld, hired as local outreach coordinator for the show, said that Simone did not have enough "background in TV production or AIDS activism" (qtd. in Kahn 66). Simone replied that "The mission of this series is not to please one constituency or another, but to provide a forum for public debate on the [AIDS] issue" (qtd. in Kahn 66).

Are we to conclude that artists can never transcend their particular epistemic boundaries? Can only those immediately involved offer valid representations? Can only women write about women, minorities about prejudice, PWAs about AIDS? Moreover, if one believes that the hegemonic culture perpetuates the power and interests of white, middle-class, heterosexual men, is it impossible for members of this group to achieve enough empathy to contribute? Are they always locked in their specific temporal realities, with everything they write suspect by those excluded?

These questions take on added significance now that AIDS seems to have plateaued among gays and shifted to heterosexuals, particularly IV drug users, their sexual partners, and their offspring. How much literary AIDS contributed to the decreasing numbers of gays newly infected cannot be measured. There will always be backsliding, with some continuing to indulge in risky behavior, but overall the campaign to educate has been successful. As the epidemic in America moves now into minority communities, new kinds of literary AIDS must be employed. To change attitudes about sex among any group is extremely difficult, no matter what teaching techniques are employed. In the case of poor, urban young people, much more than simply their lack of access to appropriate education is involved. For one thing, street codes of machismo and cool surrounding teenage sex work against the warnings and cautionary advice now being broadcast and published. For another, few people read "serious" literature any more. Another factor is economics: a number of small presses made many works of literary AIDS possible.[3] Television, film, and popular music, which have far greater potential of reaching young people, are all highly commercial and resist association with unpleasant messages. The case of Magic Johnson illustrates the problems AIDS education faces when dealing with these media. After Johnson's announcement that he was infected, media commentators immediately started to speculate whether sponsors would continue to use him in ads. If even a superstar like Magic Johnson becomes suspect once he reveals he is HIV-positive, what chance does an average artist stand?

Some analysts question how much television advertising can do. Richard L. Berke in "Can the Rich and Famous Talk America Out of Drugs?" claims that the public already sees too many famous people endorsing one product after another, so that this kind of celebrity spot does not work (E5). Surveys show that young people see themselves as too indestructible to need anyone's advice, even a celebrity's. Many in the industry feel there is only so much that television and motion pictures can do to discourage drug use and that their primary mission is to provide entertainment, not sermons. Obviously, with all the misinformation, prejudice, and reluctance to discuss sex openly that surround AIDS, the entertainment industry has even less incentive to take on HIV education, particularly when conservative voices from religion and politics strongly object to the use of explicit information about condoms. Jim Moore, an advertising official for the *Hollywood Reporter,* sums it up: "Television doesn't sit in that room to be a preacher" (qtd. in Berke E5).

As Gary Noble, assistant surgeon general and the head of the Centers for Disease Control's AIDS program commented when the government initiated a $1.8 million advertising campaign in 1990 on 8,500 network affiliate stations, "Television executives are in business to make money" (qtd. in Chase B7). All six of the public service ads were labeled "solidly mainstream" in a *Wall Street Journal* article whose headline announced: "U.S. AIDS Ads Created by WPP Seek to Highlight Risk in *Clean-Cut* Way" (19 June 1990: B7; italics mine). One, nicknamed "Sofa," shows a couple engaging in heavy petting in front of a TV, when the announcer declares, "The person you're with right now could have HIV." The young woman tries to zap the television with the remote control, but it keeps right on talking about AIDS. Available in both English and Spanish versions, the commercial features actors who could pass as either Caucasian or Hispanic. Another commercial, titled "HIV Positives," shows people of all ages and colors saying: "It's not going to happen to me." Then actual PWAs, not actors, talk about themselves. One woman is an African-American woman who says: "I got it from my husband. I didn't know he used drugs." The spot ends: "If you think you're tired of hearing about it, listen to some people who are really sick of it." Noble tried various spots on test audiences, who reacted negatively if the ads were too frightening or accusatory. "We're trying to get their attention," he said, "but fear isn't the goal" (qtd. in Chase B7). With the country deep in recession, however, will the government continue to fund such commercials?

The commercialism of the popular media not only makes it difficult for the individual artist to use the media, but indirectly contributes to the spread of the disease. Television in particular programs young people to be consumers. But slender economic opportunities, widespread racism, ghetto environments, and poor educational facilities make it next to impossible for most young persons of color to earn enough money legitimately to buy into the consumer happiness television touts. As a result, too many turn to drugs and promiscuous sex to deaden their pain, and thus put themselves at risk of contracting HIV. Those urban teenagers who do not use IV drugs or sell sex are still at greater risk because of their proximity to those who do. How does a thirteen-year-old girl from the inner city know whether the boy she agrees to have sex with hasn't shot up with a shared needle or had sex with an HIV-infected person? In spite of these greater risks, many young people continue to practice unsafe sex.

The majority of movies geared for young people tacitly condone high-risk behavior. The "cool" young adults in *About Last Night* (1986) and *Heathers* (1989), for example, have sex only a few hours after meeting one another, and even in *Casual Sex* (1988), supposedly about safe sex, prevention modes are never discussed. Although everything in the media from magazine covers to MTV encourages young people to think about sex, advertisements for condoms are rare. Mark Klein, vice president of Trojan, the nation's leading condom maker, says: "We can't get in enough markets to put together a cohesive national campaign" (qtd. in Tye 6).

Part of the problem lies with the Catholic Church's absolute condemnation of condom use, which prevents many young people from hearing about practical ways to practice safe sex. For example, John R. Dreyer, a member of the AIDS Action Committee (AAC) Massachusetts, was asked by Boston College, a Catholic school, to speak to a group of fifty young people, aged thirteen and fourteen, about AIDS. Dreyer cancelled when the College stipulated that he could not discuss the use of condoms. As Louise Rice, a registered nurse who manages HIV education for the AAC's speakers' bureau, puts it: "We make no secret of the fact that if we're asked to speak, we'll talk about condoms. We'll also talk about abstinence. We're perfectly willing to say abstinence is the most foolproof method." But she adds: "We don't go out and tell people half the story" (qtd. in Kong 19).

As AIDS shifts to young heterosexuals, they need to hear the whole story. Mircea Eliade reminds us that the modern West's privileging of "rationalism, positivism and scientism" ignores the power of myth, symbol and image over the human imagination (9–11). Because we worship science and technology, we have grown to believe that no disease can resist modern medicine. But as Allan M. Brandt emphasizes in *No Magic Bullet*, which describes how the United States fought venereal disease, only preventive measures really work. Until a vaccine can be produced—apparently still years away—art in its broadest sense—posters, TV ads, films, music—will probably be our most effective educational mode to get young people—who tend to tune out lectures and dire statistics—to practice safe sex. Artists and AIDS activists have already shown themselves willing to risk the fury of Jesse Helms and his followers by creating shockingly graphic pleas, because they know that shock is the only means of penetrating

the modern consciousness already jaded by too many commercial
assaults from mass media. The same shock tactics may be necessary to
reach inner-city youths who have tuned out traditional modes of
education.

In the early years of AIDS, gay writers combated the epidemic
through a variety of innovative and exciting literary contexts. To
combat AIDS today, artificial distinctions between high and low
types of cultural expression must be abandoned, and the power of
such forms as videos and popular music must be acknowledged. This
was recognized by Philly Bongoley Lutaaya, the popular African
singer who died of AIDS, when he used his music to educate fellow
Africans about the virus.[4]

Sadly, many African Americans are convinced that the AIDS virus
was created by whites as part of a deliberate policy of genocide, which
also includes channeling drugs into black neighborhoods and unjustly
prosecuting elected black officials. Professor Leonard Jeffries Jr. of
the City College of New York, in a speech at a cultural festival on July
20, 1991, insisted that "people called Greenberg and Weisberg and
Trigliani" are part of a "conspiracy, planned and plotted and programmed out of Hollywood" for the "destruction of black people"
(qtd. in DeParle 5). When an aide to Eugene Sawyer, the black mayor
of Chicago, claimed that Jewish doctors were infecting black babies
with AIDS, he was forced to resign. But, according to Jason DeParle,
belief in a conspiracy continues to grow, showing up on black radio,
television, books, magazines, pamphlets and poems (5). He cites a
1989 article that concluded the series on AIDS in the black paper *The
Los Angeles Sentinel* entitled "Blacks Intentionally Infected." The first
broadcast on a new public affairs show on cable's Black Entertainment
Television network was called "Black Genocide: Myth or Reality?"
And the September 1990 cover of *Essence,* a magazine with a circulation of 900,000 bore the headline, "AIDS: Is it Genocide?" DeParle
also points to John Singleton's highly successful first film *Boyz 'N the
Hood,* in which the role model father Furious Styles tells a crowd that
"they" allow crack and guns in black neighborhoods "because they
want us to kill each other off. What they couldn't do in slavery, they
are making us do to ourselves."

In discussing possible reasons why African Americans have been
reluctant to "own" AIDS, both Evelynn Hammonds, in "Race, Sex,
AIDS," and Harlon L. Dalton, in "AIDS in Blackface," cite not only
suspicion of middle-class white interference but also the desire by
African Americans to counteract stereotypes about black sexuality.[5]
Both refer to the infamous Tuskegee syphilis experiment, in which

the government deliberately withheld treatment from black male prisoners being studied (although a treatment was found halfway through) because it might have "compromised" the study. Dalton sees the conviction among many in the black community that AIDS is a deliberate policy of genocide as another reason for reluctance to own the disease or to allow needle-exchange programs in black neighborhoods. Both see white America's eagerness to accept theories that AIDS originated in Africa as one more instance of strong national racism. Sensitivity about sexual stereotypes is also seen by both as one of the causes for the strong homophobia expressed by many in the black community, another reason why many do not want to deal with the threat of AIDS. Finally, as Dalton sees it, "the uniquely problematic relationship we as a community have to the phenomenon of drug abuse complicates our dealing with AIDS" (211).

Hammonds found that most of the major publications in the black community ignored AIDS early on. *Ebony* and *Essence,* for example, did not mention it until the spring of 1987. The same was true for the official magazines of the NAACP and the National Urban League. The journal of the National Medical Association, the organization of black physicians, published a short guest editorial in late 1986, and the Atlanta-based Southern Christian Leadership Conference by that time had set up an educational program to deal with AIDS in the black community. As Hammonds puts it:

> The black media has underemphasized, though recognized, that there are significant socioeconomic cofactors in terms of the impact of AIDS in the black community. The high rate of drug use and abuse in the black community is in part a result of many other social factors—high unemployment, poor schools, inadequate housing and limited access to health care, all factors in the spread of AIDS. These affect specifically the fact that people of color with AIDS are diagnosed at more advanced stages of the disease and are dying faster. (31)

AIDS highlights the multiple problems facing persons of color in America—problems that have been centuries in the making and have no easy answers. No wonder the popular press prefers to focus on simple solutions: test all health care workers, distribute clean needles, find a magic cure. Moreover, only a handful of literary works so far have attempted to describe AIDS in persons of color, and none of these employ traditional literary modes. Perhaps the most imaginative is "The Tale of Plagues and Carnivals" (1985), by the African-American science-fiction writer Samuel R. Delany, which dramatizes AIDS devastation in the inner city among street people, who are by and large homeless drug addicts or hustlers. Delany's experimental literary mode creates a highly sophisticated and complex style that might be difficult to employ as an educational tool.

A nonfiction work giving a picture of second-phase AIDS is George Whitmore's *Someone Was Here* (1988), a journalistic account of the HIV patients at Lincoln Hospital in the South Bronx, most of whom are poor, black or Hispanic IV drug users. The perspective, however, remains that of the caregivers, not the PWAs; Whitmore, a gay, white, middle-class PWA, died in April 1989. Another which offers some perspective on the poor and minorities is the collection *AIDS: The Women,* edited by Ines Rieder and Patricia Ruppelt. Two accounts are of particular interest because they introduce voices seldom heard. One is by Marie Marthe Saint Cyr-Delpe, called "Reaching Within, Reaching Out," about AIDS in the Haitian community. The other is by Lynn Hampton. Written in street language, "Hookers with AIDS— the Search" details Hampton's attempts to get prostitutes in Atlanta to have their clients use condoms.

Dominique Lapierre's *Beyond Love* (1991), a book almost totally about whites involved with AIDS, is indicative of the multiple stereo- types and prejudice surrounding minority persons with AIDS. In one brief scene, Lapierre tacitly reinforces existing prejudices when he distinguishes between drug users and homosexuals. He intro- duces a black nurse, Gloria Taylor, whom he describes in a stereotypical manner: "With her generous bosom, her unaltering smile, and her Southern accent, she was like a black character from an antebellum plantation." He then quotes her: "Drug addicts were very different in character from homosexuals. They denied their illness. To them, only one thing counted: getting their drug allowance. If you said to them 'That syringe will kill you,' they would answer: 'I couldn't give a damn. I'll take that risk' " (316). Lapierre echoes Taylor's distinction between the types of PWAs, writing that "the slaves of hard drugs were a class apart" (317). What emerges are vivid class distinctions between the well-educated, white, middle-class gays, who learn as much about their disease as possible and often know more about it than those caring for them, and the lower-class, black and Hispanic IV drug users who live only for the next fix and come across as people totally defined by their addiction rather than as individual- ized human beings. Such reductive characterizations only reinforce existing stereotypes which dominate our racist society. All white gays are not polite and well educated. All IV drug users are not suicidal. And it is just as reifying to perceive all drug users by their addiction as it is to perceive all gays through their sexual preference. Samuel

Jackson's brilliant portrayal of the crack addict Gator in Spike Lee's film *Jungle Fever* presents a much more humanized picture of people who do drugs. Mario Van Peebles's *New Jack City* also makes the drug lord Nino Brown, played by Wesley Snipes, much more complex than the two-dimensional villains who usually populate gangster films.

The multiple racist and homophobic stereotypes hounding gay African Americans are highly destructive as Melvin Dixon clearly delineates. In his novel *Vanishing Rooms* (1991), the gay black narrator is taunted by sadistic Italian toughs who later kill his white lover: "'He a black nigger faggot, yeah, he a faggot, a nigger, too,' and shouting and laughing so close they made acid out of every bit of safety I thought we had. Now their hate had eaten up everything" (15).

Marlon Riggs's film *Tongues Untied*, which garnered virulent criticism from the extreme right when shown on PBS, attempts in a highly stylized way to counteract the anguish engendered by the hate gay blacks experience not only from whites but from a large proportion of the African-American community. Riggs shows the sensitive tenderness and joyous sensuality of gay black men loving one another. The poet and performance artist Essex Hemphill, who recently edited a collection of writings by African Americans, *Brother to Brother* (1991), many of which deal with AIDS, is one of the outstanding cast. However, possibly because of the film's expressionistic style, I found its references to AIDS muted, perhaps deliberately so, compared to its strong appeal for tolerance and understanding for a group doubly marginalized in our society. Also, I question how many young persons at risk were watching it. I suspect it reached primarily an already converted audience, although its value as a positive affirmation of identity for gay blacks cannot be overestimated. I believe, however, that to reach many of the young persons of color at risk, works which possess the strong appeal of Singleton's *Boyz 'N the Hood* are needed.

Because many people today are asking what constitutes American culture, questions of how to achieve a fair balance in a multicultural society problematize responsible representation of AIDS. Moreover, fear in 1991 of health care workers transmitting the virus, after the Florida dentist David Acer somehow infected five of his patients, has shifted much attention away from the need for effective educational strategies to questions of rights and possible punitive legislation. Nevertheless, I am convinced that the most effective way of reaching young people is not through grim preaching and statistics but through the forms of entertainment they love—movies, television, and music.

In 1989 I attended a conference with the optimistic title "Restoring American Education," where Houston Baker, Albert M. Greenfield Professor of Human Relations and director of the Center for Black Literature and Culture at the University of Pennsylvania, debated the topic "Upper Crust Dead White Men; or, Whither the Study of Western Civilization?" Replying to why Johnny and Jonetta cannot read, Baker said that instead of following Allan Bloom's suggestion that we try to wean young people away from the pleasant but repetitious sexuality of rock music, perhaps we should start listening to the lyrics of the currently popular rap music. It is difficult for me, I admit, to get past the raw anger and adolescent braggadocio in much of this music to estimate what its potential for AIDS education might be, especially since the contention that its hostility focuses on the hegemonic culture is only partially true. Women, sex, and family are often treated in a highly cavalier, macho manner befitting the "cool" outlaw image to which much of this music aspires. The one rap album that has garnered the most opprobrium, 2 Live Crew's *As Nasty as They Wanna Be,* glorifies in obscene language savage treatment of women. Henry Louis Gates, Jr., chairman of African-American Studies at Harvard, argued at the trial of a record dealer in Florida that such language was actually used for humorous, ironic purposes that parallel the intention in other African-American oral traditions. I agree with Gates and others who question why only 2 Live Crew and other black rappers are being hounded, while Madonna can simulate masturbation with a crucifix on stage and make millions, and Andrew Dice Clay can ridicule women, gays, and blacks in sewer language and become a sought-after concert and film star. The larger question, though, is how much potential does this music have to teach young people about the risks of AIDS? Ultimately, I have come to believe that rap has great potential if its artists determine to wage all-out war against AIDS. With its strong use of parody and street language, its lack of the usual plot and continuities of popular lyrics, rap is the street's version of postmodernism, and young people listen to it. I can only hope that everyone in the entertainment industry devoted to pleasing young people will also devote themselves to keeping them alive.

As Timothy F. Murphy, co-editor of *Writing AIDS,* points out, questions about AIDS are "solvable only by rethinking our society."[6] That AIDS is becoming more and more concentrated among poor, urban, African Americans exacerbates already dangerous divisions in our culture. The prominence of divisive rhetoric in the 1992 presidential campaign presages heightening racist tensions in a country that has yet to come to terms with its multicultural identity. AIDS is only one of the many problems threatening America. Our educational system, with the exception of our graduate schools, is failing. Our health care-delivery system leaves many without basic medical attention. Our cities are no longer proud centers of beauty and culture, but dangerous warrens of crime. Our former world leadership as an industrial power has seriously declined, as Germany and Japan have surpassed us in the ability to develop affordable, reliable consumer items. And we are so far losing the war against AIDS because those who are supposed to lead refuse to admit the seriousness of this epidemic. Those in the trenches have had to be their own leaders, and they have done a superb job in trying to arouse a sleeping nation to the mounting danger. But perhaps we need to rethink our national priorities. Can we afford to fight more wars over oil when our educational and health care systems are failing? There is fierce anger in America at the perceived unwillingness of national leadership to try to redress the many problems confronting us. AIDS is only one of these problems, but its grim nature symbolizes the potential disintegration of our culture if we do not take definite steps toward restoring it to good health.

Notes

1. For a deconstructive analysis of literary AIDS, see Edelman, "The Plague of Discourse."

2. In a later full-length work entitled *AIDS: the Facts,* Langone reaffirms his position, writing in the chapter "How Easily Is AIDS Transmitted between Men and Women?" that although "anonymous sexual contact, heterosexual as well as homosexual, is, as they say, akin to playing Russian roulette," this does "not necessarily mean the roulette game is the same as when it is played with dirty, shared needles, or by a male who is the receiving partner in unprotected anal sex. AIDS is now, and is likely to be for some time, largely spread by certain well-defined forms of behavior, perhaps helped along by certain conditions and circumstances; and vaginal sex is not now, and may never be, high among them, at least not in the United States" (84).

3. In 1984, Gay Sunshine Press published Paul Reed's *Facing It,* and Knights Press published Daniel Curzon's *The World Can Break Your Heart.* Other works about AIDS published by Knights Press include the following: David Rees's *The Wrong Apple* (1987); Geoff Mains's *Gentle Warriors* (1988); Clayton R. Graham's [Larry Ebmeier] *Tweeds* (1987); Joel Redon's *Bloodstream* (1989); Jeff Black's *Gardy and Erin* (1989); Tim Barrus's *Genocide* (1989); and the short story collection by Chris Davis, *The Boys in the Bars* (1989), which contains several dealing with

AIDS. After 1987, with the publication of Randy Shilts's *And the Band Played On* by St. Martin's Press, more mainstream publishers responded. St. Martin's Press also published Christopher Davis's novel *Valley of the Shadow* (1988) and Joel Redon's *If Not on Earth, Then in Heaven* (1991). Crown also responded well: in addition to *Poets for Life* (1989), they published Robert Ferro's novel *Second Son* (1988); Holly Uyemoto's *Rebel Without a Clue* (1989), and Paul Monette's two AIDS novels, *Afterlife* (1990) and *Halfway Home* (1991). Harper published M. E. Kerr's *Night Kites* (1987), John Weir's *The Irreversible Decline of Eddie Socket* (1989), and Armistead Maupin's *Tales of the City* series, beginning with *Baby Cakes* (1984) and concluding with *Sure of You* (1989). The annotated bibliography gives complete publication information on these titles.

4. "The AIDS Quarterly" featured Lutaaya in a ninety-minute show called "Born in Africa." PBS rebroadcast it in a sixty-minute version, shown in the Boston area on December 17, 1991.

5. Professor Houston Baker, Albert M. Greenfield Professor of Human Relations and Director of Black Literature and Culture at the University of Pennsylvania, kindly brought these two articles to my attention.

6. Murphy, assistant professor of Philosophy in the Biomedical Sciences at the University of Illinois in Chicago, offered this observation while reviewing the manuscript of this article.

Works Cited

Baldwin, James. "James Baldwin: Price of a Ticket." PBS's *American Masters* series, August 1989.

Bateson, Mary Catherine, and Richard Goldsby. *Thinking AIDS: The Social Response to the Biological Threat.* Reading, Mass.: Addison-Wesley, 1988.

Berke, Richard L. "Can the Rich and Famous Talk America Out of Drugs?" *New York Times* 12 Nov. 1989: E5.

Bram, Christopher. *In Memory of Angel Clare.* New York: Donald I. Fine, 1989.

Brandt, Allan M. *No Magic Bullet: A Social History of Venereal Disease in the United States.* New York: Oxford University Press, 1985.

Buckley, William F. "Identify All the Carriers." *New York Times* 18 Mar. 1986: A27.

Chase, Marilyn. "U.S. AIDS Ads Created by WPP Unit Seek to Highlight Risk in Clean-Cut Way." *Wall Street Journal* 19 June 1990: B7.

Dalton, Harlon L. "AIDS in Blackface." *Daedalus* 118.3 (Summer 1989): 205–27.

Delany, Samuel R. "Appendix A: The Tale of Plagues and Carnivals; or, Some Informal Remarks toward the Modular Calculus, Part Five," *Flight from Nevèrÿon.* New York: Bantam Books, 1985.

DeParle, Jason. "For Some Blacks, Social Ills Seem to Follow White Plans." *New York Times* 11 Aug. 1991: E5.

Dixon, Melvin. *Vanishing Rooms.* New York: E. P. Dutton, 1991.

Edelman, Lee. "The Plague of Discourse: Politics, Literary Theory, and AIDS." *Displacing Homophobia: Gay Male Perspectives in Literature and Culture.* Ed.

Ronald R. Butters, John M. Clum, and Michael Moon. Durham, N.C.: Duke University Press, 1989: 289–305.

Eliade, Mircea. *Images and Symbols. Studies in Religious Symbolism.* Trans. Philip Mairet. New York: Sheed & Ward, 1961.

Gambone, Philip. "Anyplace Gay, USA." *Bay Windows* 18 Jan. 1990: 16.

Grant, Daniel. "Artists' Insurance Suffers from AIDS Assumption." *Boston Herald* 30 Nov. 1989: 74.

Grover, Jan Zita. "AIDS Culture." *Women's Review of Books* 6.7 (April 1989): 5–6.

Hammonds, Evelynn. "Race, Sex, AIDS: The Construction of 'Other.' " *Radical America* 20.6 (November/December 1987): 28–36.

Hemphill, Essex, ed. *Brother to Brother.* Boston: Alyson Publications, 1991.

Kahn, Joseph P. " 'AIDS Quarterly' draws angry reactions." *Boston Globe* 17 Oct. 1989: 63.

Kimmelman, Michael. "Bitter Harvest: AIDS and the Arts." *New York Times* 19 Mar. 1989: H1.

Kong, Dolores. "Speaker cancels BC AIDS talk." *Boston Globe* 19 July 1991: 15.

Langone, John. "AIDS." *Discover* December 1985: 28–53.

———. *AIDS: the Facts.* Boston: Little, Brown, 1988.

Lapierre, Dominique. *Beyond Love.* New York: Warner Books, 1991.

Leavitt, David. "Fears That Haunt a Scrubbed America." *New York Times* 19 Aug. 1990: H1.

———. *The Lost Language of Cranes.* New York: Alfred A. Knopf, 1986.

———. *A Place I've Never Been.* New York: Viking, 1990.

———. "The Way I Live Now." *New York Times Magazine* 9 July 1989: 28.

Loewenstein, Sophia Freud. "Troubled times." *Women's Review of Books* 7.20 (July 1990): 22.

Monette, Paul. *Afterlife.* New York: Crown Publications, 1990.

———. *Halfway Home.* New York: Crown Publications, 1991.

Murphy, Timothy F., and Suzanne Poirier, eds. *Writing AIDS: Gay Literature, Language and Analysis.* New York: Columbia University Press, 1993.

Rieder, Ines, and Patricia Ruppelt, eds. *AIDS: The Women.* Pittsburgh: Cleis Press, 1988.

Schulman, Sarah. *People in Trouble.* New York: E. P. Dutton, 1990.

Singer, Linda. "Bodies—Pleasures—Powers." *Differences: A Journal of Feminist Cultural Studies* 1 (1989): 45–65.

Sontag, Susan. *Illness as Metaphor.* New York: Farrar, Straus and Giroux, 1978.

———. *AIDS and Its Metaphors.* New York: Farrar, Straus and Giroux, 1989.

———. "The Way We Live Now." *The New Yorker* 24 Nov. 1986: 42–51.

Treichler, Paula A. "AIDS, Homophobia and Biomedical Discourse: An Epidemic of Signification." *Cultural Studies* 1 (1988): 263–305.

Trilling, Lionel. "Manners, Morals, and the Novel." *The Liberal Imagination.* New York: Viking Press, 1950.

Tye, Larry. "Drive to encourage US to use condoms against AIDS stalls." *Boston Globe* 22 July 1991: 1.

Vendler, Helen. "Feminism and Literature." *The New York Review of Books* 31 May 1990: 19–25.

Whitmore, George. *Someone Was Here: Profiles in the AIDS Epidemic.* New York: St. Martin's Press, 1988.

AIDS Writing and the Creation of a Gay Culture

In the Preface to *The Birth Of The Clinic* Michel Foucault writes: "It may well be that we belong to an age of criticism whose lack of a primary philosophy reminds us at every moment of its reign and its fatality: an age of intelligence that keeps us irremediably at a distance from an original language. . . . We are doomed historically to history, to the patient construction of discourses about discourses and to the task of hearing what has already been said" (xv–xvi).

It is perhaps unfair to continue an argument with a man after he is dead, but it is increasingly necessary and I doubt Foucault would have minded, especially considering the gusto he displayed in late night discussions about this issue of primary discourse in our time, specifically the emergence of the possibility of such a thing as gay culture and its corollary, gay literature. I would not presume to try to reproduce Foucault's subtle—and, to my mind, shifting—position on this topic; for my part, this despair about primary discourse seemed to me a result of the commanding position the academic mind has achieved in our culture, reigning over the recording and evaluation of the activity of intelligence in general. The academic mind, I argued, looks out and sees reflections of itself and its interior processes, not the world as it is happening around us. We are doomed not historically but academically to the patient construction of discourses about discourses, to the task of hearing what has already been said. History dooms us to something else altogether.

Acknowledging the enormous loss to this discussion caused by Foucault's death from AIDS, I would like to try to extend this argument to the extraordinary surge of writing that has been occasioned by the advent of the AIDS epidemic, acts of primary discourse whose nature, depth, and value seem to me in danger of being obscured by the natural bent of the academic mind. It is noticeable that secondary discourses about AIDS—how the media speaks when it speaks about AIDS, studies of the metaphors used in AIDS discussions—naturally float to the surface of academic journals or serve as the occasion for thematic issues, while the primary acts of speech uttered in confrontation with the thing itself are neglected or misunderstood.

What history dooms us to is the shock of events, happenings that break over us and challenge the human spirit to give back an answer—"answering back the hammer-blows of Fortune," in the words of the final chorus of the *Antigone*. This urge to answer back, to declare one's presence even at the cost of acknowledging the original blow to the spirit, lies at the very heart of what we mean by culture, that shared collection of individual acts of the spirit that articulate who we are and how we find ourselves in this life.

History dooms us to the shock of events, and an epidemic is a historical event, the unleashing of an infectious—in this case, lethal—disease in a population. AIDS is not a condition to be managed, like high blood pressure or poverty. AIDS is not just a disease, like cancer or sickle-cell anemia. AIDS is not a chronic medical state, like diabetes—though it may become one. AIDS in our time is an *event*, a calamity, like a forest fire, like the blitz of London. AIDS is an epidemic and an epidemic is an event.

More precisely, an epidemic is the occurrence of death as a social event. Usually death is one of the most individualizing and private experiences a person can undergo. But death is sometimes a social event, a shared reality; it was so in the trenches of World War I, in the gas chambers of Auschwitz, in the killing fields of Cambodia. When death becomes a social event, the individual death is both robbed of its utter privacy and uniquely individual meaning and simultaneously amplified with the resonance of social significance and historical consequence. When death is a social event, both the individual *and the community* are threatened with irreparable loss.

An epidemic is a shared social disaster played out on the bodies of the afflicted. AIDS, of course, is not a gay disease. But, given the means of transmission, AIDS managed to gain momentum and achieve epidemic force first in the gay community. As John Preston has said, "AIDS is not a gay disease. . . . It is, however, a catastrophe for gay men" (4). Although it has ravaged other individuals (hemophiliacs, transfusion recipients) and diverse social groups (Haitians, Africans, IV drug users and, through them, the mostly black and Hispanic inner-city underclass, and—soon—American teenagers), it was the happenstance of history that the disease should first achieve epidemic proportions in the gay community. This was to have severe consequences both for the world and for the gay community. The world, motivated by a disastrous combination of prejudice, vicious self-righteousness, murderous indifference to the fate of a group mistakenly thought to be "other," and massive, panicked denial, ignored the problem and blindly allowed the epidemic to get out of control, with grim consequences that have not even begun to be perceived, much less tallied. For the gay community, it meant that the AIDS epidemic was to become the central fact of its history at this moment, as elemental an event for this fledgling community as the Holocaust was for Jews all over the world.

I

It is clear now that the history of the liberated gay community in America is divided into two phases. First was the original act of constitution as a self-acknowledged community, initiated by the Stonewall Riots in June 1969 and unfolded in the seventies when a vast act of social transformation reshaped the lives and attitudes of millions of Americans—a social event of such magnitude that it can only be compared to the half-century-old civil rights movement—but which has characteristically received virtually no attention from our so-called social scientists. The second phase commenced with the advent of the AIDS epidemic at the beginning of the eighties, an event that threatened to destroy this community both physically and spiritually.

The initial shock at this dawning social disaster was compounded by the peculiar relations of the gay community to the surrounding society, which has always favored resounding silence as the most effective means of gay repression. Thus, when gay men found themselves in the middle of a social catastrophe, found themselves and their friends wasting away from an unknown but clearly rapidly spreading disease, their panic was compounded by the hostility of the Reagan political regime, the indifference of the national medical establishment, and the virtual silence of the media. The shameful silence of the *New York Times,* the nation's self-proclaimed "newspaper of record" as well as the hometown paper for the city that was the epicenter of this catastrophe, left gay New Yorkers in a near schizophrenic situation: on the one hand, friends were falling ill left and right, life became a surrealistic series of medical disasters, hospital vigils, and memorial services; on the other hand, everyday life went on as if nothing were happening, the media were nearly silent, and straight friends and co-workers, going about their normal lives, seemed to be living on some other planet. "It was as if a war was going on in our city," said William M. Hoffman, "and half the city was in rubble, but people weren't mentioning it" (qtd. in Kaufman 14).

Piling the insult of silence on top of the grotesque injuries wreaked by AIDS left the gay community in a state of political confusion and spiritual despair, for the impact of any social disaster is mute until it is articulated in words, reflected in the imagination. Only then do we realize what is happening to us; only when we can relive in the imagination what has happened to us in life does it become real for us. As Hannah Arendt observed, "The impact of factual reality, like all other human experiences, needs speech if it is to survive the moment of experience, needs talk and communication with others to remain sure of itself" (495). It is for precisely this reason that gay writers became pivotal players in the second act of gay history.

During the first decade of gay liberation, the community itself seemed to undergo a process of spontaneous transubstantiation: when the drag queens and the boys in the bars initiated it all by fighting back, it was as if a signal went out, heard by all, calling everyone to the colors. The process of transformation ignited everywhere, and the enormously complex act of redefinition—sexually, politically, morally, psychologically, interpersonally, spiritually—was spontaneous, decentralized, and multiple. Something akin to Nietzsche's "transvaluation of all values" was happening all over the place. This enormous ferment unleashed in 1969 gained velocity during the seventies, creating new social spaces, new relationships, new institutions, even new sexual acts, and igniting the imaginations of the first generation of gay writers, who emerged in the late seventies avid to reflect in their writing these fundamental changes that were already clearly sweeping through our lives.

With the advent of AIDS in the early eighties a new and heavier task fell to the writers: the job of sounding the alarm, mobilizing the community both politically and spiritually, delineating the shape of this disaster breaking over us, and initiating the discourse of AIDS in the face of the silence of the national media and institutionalized medicine. It is notable that it was a gay newspaper, *The New York Native,* that first announced the existence of this disease—before the Centers for Disease Control did—by insisting that a handful of cases of a rare cancer must be connected to the unheard-of pneumonia that was striking people down.[1] It was Larry Kramer's famous 1983 essay in the *Native,* "1,112 and Counting" which swept away the confusion and mobilized gay people from one end of the American continent to the other.

Taken completely by surprise, enraged and demoralized by what seemed like a malevolent symbolism in a disease that not only appeared to target gay men but that seemed to zero in on sexual activity, the locus of most of the hard-won liberation of the previous decade, the gay community reeled. One of the first to confront the panic, conflict, and grief that the sudden appearance of this new and almost unbeliev-able disease engendered was William Hoffman in his play *As Is.* "Personally, I was trying to cope with the death of friends—four in particular at the time—and the illness around me," he said (qtd. in Kaufman 14). At almost the same time, Larry Kramer, furious at the inaction of the gay community, the medical establishment, and politi-cal "leaders" from city hall to the White House, took to the stage with *The Normal Heart,* an intensely political play that rang out with a stinging indictment of official indifference and a near-maddened call to arms.

As the epidemic expanded, as more people fell ill and died, as visits to the hospital and the funeral home became regular, if bizarre, social occasions for gay men, the community moved into life in the war zone. Like other gay men in major urban areas, gay writers spent an increasing amount of time caring for the ill; confronted by the epidemic every which way they turned, it began to seem the only serious thing to write about. Robert Ferro's novel *Second Son* was written while the author, ill himself, was caring for his dying lover, and published only months before his own death from AIDS. In his novel *Valley of the Shadow,* Christopher David sought to present the human reality behind the impersonal—and increasingly frequent—obituaries of young gay men appearing in the newspapers. This first-person fiction was a courageous act of imagination and sustained with remarkable beauty a clear-eyed depiction of the grief, loss, and love that would soon become common throughout the gay world.

Randy Shilts, determined to set down the objective record so long ignored by the media, produced *And the Band Played On,* a massive, relentless, hypnotic, and epic narrative of the first five years of the AIDS epidemic that laid bare the unfolding politics and history of this disaster with such persuasive force and detailed accumulation of fact that the book itself became a political event. Paul Monette, seeking to make personal sense of the holocaust that had swept over his life, wrote *Borrowed Time,* in which he etched with passion and anger the impact of AIDS on two lovers, while his great poem cycle, *Love Alone,* raised a shattering paean to the death of a whole genera-tion of gay men, "the story that endlessly eludes the decorum of the press" (xii).

George Whitmore learned of his own illness while writing *Someone*

Was Here, a book of personal reportage in which he managed, before his death, to show people with AIDS (PWAs) as the concrete individuals they were, not just statistics and categories, and not just gay men. At the same time, his friend Victor Bumbalo was working on "Adam and the Experts", a play about their friendship during the crisis. "Writing the play was a painful experience," Bumbalo told an interviewer, "but also very, very cathartic."

"Did you have to wait a long time after your friend died to be able to write it?" he was asked.

"No, he was alive when I finished it. He read the play. This was George Whitmore. We talked about it, and he loved the idea of the play. And then he said an interesting thing to me. He asked me, 'Is Eddie going to die during the play?' And I said, 'No, I don't think so,' because I was nervous and trying to avoid it. He said, 'Then, as a PWA, I would be very uncomfortable watching your play; it would be denying what may happen to me.' "

"And what did he say when he read the play?" asked the interviewer.

"He really like the play a lot. But then, George is George; he's also a writer. So first, of course, he had his emotional experience with it, and then he looked at it as a writer. I mean, I was writing this play and he was writing *Someone Was Here.* We were two of the most depressed people in New York!" (O'Conner 87).

Around this time, according to Andrew Holleran, "there came a strange point—this was years into the epidemic—when I realized that all the writing that was not about AIDS that I myself was reading seemed so irrelevant and pointless, that it really was like playing bridge while the Titanic was sinking. It just was impossible to talk about anything else" (15). Holleran's monthly essays in *Christopher Street Magazine,* collected in *Ground Zero,* became like new paths of thought through the wilderness that life with AIDS had become, probing, exploring, grieving the past, mapping the way we live now.

Robert Patrick's searing one-act comedy *Pouf Positive,* printed in *Untold Decade: Seven Comedies of Gay Romance,* was a final gift to an ex-lover whose last request the author found on his answering machine when he returned to the city after the man's death: "You ask if you can do anything for me, Robert? Yes, write a comedy about this absurd mess." And Harvey Fierstein, in his comic trilogy *Safe Sex,* explored the new social conundrums AIDS has established with a rare blend of wit and anger.

Larry Kramer weighed in yet again with his *Reports from the holocaust,* a collection of passionate essays and thunderous calls to action that proved just how mighty the pen can be—not since Émile

Zola's *"J'Accuse"* has the sheer power inherent in the written word been used with such polemical skill and political impact.

In *Personal Dispatches,* John Preston, who had stopped writing for over a year after he was diagnosed, found a way out of his own panic and despair by collecting essays from some twenty writers who had to put their personal and professional agendas on hold and turn to the written word to confront the plague that increasingly threatened their circle of friends, their lovers, their own bodies. "The drive of each author was to bear witness," said Preston in an interview, "and in rereading the book, I was struck by how often that word was used. . . . and the word 'witness' is not a passive word, it's a very active verb. To 'witness' is not simply to make note, not simply to record, although there is a power in that. It is to go out and see what is going on" (qtd. in Pettit 43).

Two of the contributors to Preston's anthology died before the book could be printed. And well over half of all these writers mentioned are seropositive, ill, or already dead.

These writers—and many others[2] I have not mentioned—registered the initial shock of AIDS as a historical event, that moment when a deep shudder seized the soul of the gay community. Because of criminal neglect and indifference, this eminently preventable epidemic, which should have been treated as an emergency but was not, spread throughout the land and became a medical fact and an omnipresent threat. By the late eighties the emergency had become a condition of life, particularly for gay men. "We seem to have reached a plateau of some sort," commented Holleran in 1988, "in which people have adapted to it in a strange way. . . . It's a way of life now" (qtd. in Jack 21).

A way of life that Paul Monette, who continued to be able to write against all odds, explored in two further novels:

> "It's never going to be over, is it?" asked Mark, not really expecting an answer.
> "Someday. Not for us."
> "Will anyone understand what it was like?" It was curiously easy, perched on the mountain of death, to speak about the future when all of them would be gone.
> "Maybe the gay ones will."
> "Yeah, but they'll have to see through all the lies. 'Cause history's just white folks covering their ass." (*Afterlife* 264)

Beyond even anger and grief, gay writers realized they now stood in the full noon of disaster, unrelenting, unending, inevitable; and, like Michael Lassell in his great poem "How to Watch Your Brother Die," they set down a record to stand against the lies. Peter McGeehee, in his two extraordinary novels *Boys Like Us* and *Sweetheart,* describes what life is like when you live amidst a circle of friends, an elective family, that you know is soon going to disappear, when imminent absence is a palpable, felt pressure affecting every present moment. It was his great achievement to wrest comedy from material saturated with such intense mortality.

Edmund White too described the new situation with a precise clarity:

"Mark thought this summer everything was just as it had been the twelve preceding summers. The only thing different was that this summer would end the series.

"He wanted to know how to enjoy these days without clasping them so tightly he'd stifle the pleasure. But he didn't want to drug himself on the moment either and miss out on what was happening to him. He was losing his best friend, the witness to his life. The skill for enjoying a familiar pleasure about to disappear was hard to acquire. ... Knowing how to appreciate the rhythms of these last casual moments—to cherish them while letting them stay casual—demanded a new way of navigating time" ("Palace Days" 164).

This growing body of work defining the face of AIDS, limning it in our public and collective imagination, seems to me more than a literary accomplishment. These are individual acts of language performed in the full light of the community's crisis. They are, I would argue, the primary discourse of AIDS, a public dialogue that articulates the experience of the community and constitutes, beyond the shadow of a doubt, the creation of a culture. This new writing is not "discourses about discourses"; indeed, it was impelled into being by the urgent necessity to put speech where there had been cultural silence, for in our present circumstances, as the motto of ACT UP succinctly puts it, "Silence = Death." The task was not to "hear what has already been said" but to utter the new word, the word that would reveal what was happening to us and, at the same time, would constitute our answer, our response, our resistance.

This writing lays before us an example of a living culture, culture as a spontaneous act, for culture is a complex social event that creates the public space in which a community comes into being through participation. Generally, we tend to think of culture either objectively, from the outside, as an anthropologist might look at Samoa, or passively, as a tradition that's there, that is somehow fundamental and undergirds our intellectual life today. But we are not outside this culture that is ours, we have no disinterested Archimedian point of view from which to study it; we *are* the Samoans. Nor is culture any longer a tradition handed down to us, shoved at us by the previous generation; indeed, a great portion of the cultural activity of the last century has centered on the collapse of this tradition and its consequences. Insofar as it exists today, culture is an event that requires activity at both ends, on the part of the initiator who raises a voice to speak, and on the part of the hearer who actively attends to the word. Culture *is* the relationship between these two, and that relationship is an activity, of speaking and of attending, and that activity creates the bond that is what we mean by the word *community*.

II

The writing that is emerging from the AIDS crisis is, to my mind, startlingly different from our normal understanding of writing and books in this society—that is, writing as a literary career or profession, on the one hand, and books as a commercial commodity and the object of aesthetic appreciation, on the other. Virtually all the writers I know of who have grappled with AIDS in their work have experienced this as an interruption in their career.[3] They speak of putting aside their personal agendas to care for friends, to do political or volunteer work, to manage their own illness, and finally to confront this disaster with the tools of their trade, to use the imagination and the capacities of language and its forms to comprehend what is happening.

"Many of the contributors to [Personal Dispatches] are activists," said Preston. "They are doing things that must be done. There's a quote at the beginning of the book, 'For some of us must storm the castles. Some define the happening,' that I hesitated before using because it seemed to imply a separation of roles. Writing on the one hand, action on the other. I kept it in because I came to understand that it was a corporate statement; that both must be done and that much of it is done by the same people" (qtd. in Pettit 43).

"Write as if you were dying," admonished Annie Dillard in the 28 May 1989 *New York Times Book Review,* evidently not imagining that a whole generation of gay writers might be. "At the same time," she added, "assume you write for an audience consisting solely of terminal patients" (1). When this is actually the case, profession and career do not begin to define or situate the activity of writing.

"The purpose of AIDS writing," declared Preston, "has to be

found outside of any conventions that contemporary criticism and publishing might try to impose on us. The canons are proven to be ineffective, inappropriate. What is 'literature' becomes a meaningless academic question when what is defined can't accommodate what is happening in our lives. . . . Those of us who are writing about AIDS can't worry about these definitions any more. We can't be concerned with careerism, with academic acceptance, or with having the fashions of the day dictate how we write. We can now only deal with being witnesses" ("AIDS Writing").

The poems in *Love Alone* that coursed out of Paul Monette in the months immediately following his lover's death were not conceived as a literary strategy. "Writing them quite literally kept me alive," said the author, "for the only time I wasn't wailing and trembling was when I was hammering at these poems" (xii). When Randy Shilts took a leave of absence from his job as an investigative reporter to write *And the Band Played On,* he intended to change the world, to shock the country into taking action that would end the epidemic. That all he achieved was another book, albeit a best-seller, does not alter the original intention; indeed, the sardonic, even bitter, tone with which he recounted in *Esquire* magazine the story of the book's success and his own utter failure starkly reveals his original intention (Shilts, "Talking").

If it is an inescapable irony for the artist that acts of the spirit, when put into the world, immediately become transformed into exchange commodities—for instance, books to be sold and bought— still, this does not change either the author's original intention or the work's essence. In fact, it only creates more paradoxes. "Who wants to read this fiction?" asked Allen Barnett, whose harrowing stories remind us that reading is sometimes a courageous act; "It hurts me to re-read them" (personal communication). "My fear is these works are going to die in the studio," said Kenneth Lithgow, who has produced some of the most powerful depictions of AIDS on canvas I know of: "People see them and cry. Who would want to live with these paintings?" (qtd. in Kaufman 18). And Holleran writes of books about AIDS, "I really don't know who reads them for pleasure" (*Ground Zero* 12).

Aesthetic appreciation is neither the intention nor the relevant response to such works. "I don't consider myself an artist," writes Larry Kramer. "I consider myself a very opinionated man who uses words as fighting tools. I perceive certain wrongs that make me very angry, and somehow I hope that if I string my words together with enough skill, people will hear them and respond. I am under no delusion that this will necessarily be the case, but I seem to have no choice but to try" (*Reports* 145). And Paul Monette says of *Love Alone,* "I would rather have this volume filed under AIDS than under Poetry, because if these words speak to anyone they are for those who are mad with loss, to let them know they are not alone" (xi). Whatever it is, this writing is not about the making of well-wrought urns.

What distinguishes this AIDS writing from other literary production in our time is not only the writers' intention but the unique situation in which the act of writing occurs. This is not strong emotion recollected in tranquility; these are reports from the combat zone. AIDS writing is urgent; it is engaged and activist writing; it is writing in response to a present threat; it is in it, of it, and aims to affect it. I can think of no good parallel for this in literary history. As far as I know, most of the writing done about the Holocaust was published after 1945, when the nightmare was over in reality and began to haunt the imagination. And while the closest parallel might be the poetry that came out of the trenches of the first World War, the bulk of that writing was published, reviewed and read after the war; whereas this AIDS writing is not only being produced in the trenches, as it were, but is being published, read by its public and evaluated by the critics in the midst of the crisis. It is as if Sassoon's poetry were being mimeographed in the trenches and distributed to be read by men under fire—the immediacy of these circumstances precludes the possibility of this being a merely aesthetic enterprise. The aesthetic requires distance and the distance is not available, not to the writer, not to the reader.

Because of this peculiarity, the truth or beauty—that is, the inherent excellence—of this writing will not wait upon posterity for judgment. In this onrush of death, posterity—even posterity as an imagined frame for the activity of writing—is a luxury. The time is not available. Writers who are facing death are writing for an audience that is dying. Never could I have imagined ten years ago hearing regular discussions from writers about whether they would live long enough to finish a project. Never could I have imagined feeling, on a normal basis, this terrible urgency to get the book out while the author is still alive.

"During the year after Roger died," Paul Monette told an interviewer, "I wrote my book of poems and I spent the next eight or nine months writing the book *Borrowed Time,* assuming I would be dead in a year. I felt that I should get up in the morning and write the best I could that day and put it to bed that night, for who knew what would happen the next day. It was a sense of urgency, a calamitous urgency throughout the writing of those two books" (qtd. in Stomberg 19).

Many artists and art movements in the twentieth century have tried to shake themselves loose from the deadening context of posterity-as-judge, to avoid the spectre of the eternal museum outside time to which art is consigned, in order to free the creative act and its inherent energy. It is a terrible irony that for gay writers AIDS has knocked to smithereens all such constraining cultural frameworks.

A comparison may make clearer the unparalleled circumstances in which this work is being written. Anne Frank's diary, which might at first be thought a good literary parallel, had its own special beauty; but, on the one hand, it was written without her really knowing what would happen, and, on the other hand, we read it knowing there is nothing we can do about the course of events. But AIDS writing is about something we know *is* happening, *now,* and about which we must in fact *do* something. Of necessity this writing arises from the moment and intends to have its impact in the present. As Sarah Pettit has pointed out, what is "wholly different about the present sort of bearing witness is that it's witnessing *in the midst* of the nightmare. Speaking out in the midst of an event has to hold with it the notion that witnessing can effect change" (43).

John Preston agrees: "The purpose of AIDS writing now is *to get it all down.* The purpose of the writer in the time of AIDS is *to bear witness.* . . . To live in a time of AIDS and to understand what is going on, *writing must be action. Writing must be accompanied by action. Writing is not what our teachers told us, something that stands alone.*

"To be a writer in the time of AIDS is to be a truth-teller. The truth is more horrible than anything people want to hear. . . . The truth is devastating. The truth can't be contained in a pleasantly structured short story that will satisfy the readers of a literary magazine." ("AIDS Writing")

III

"This writing about AIDS reports from the thing itself. It unsettles all the assumptions culture codified about how art is supposed to work and how long it is supposed to take for it to work and who decides whether what is working is really art," writes Robert Dawidoff in *Personal Dispatches.* "The reader and writer community of AIDS has rediscovered the roots of any kind of writing, the roots in human survival, expression, ritual and need. We need to have these things written. The information, the truth, the anger, the philosophy, the history, the fiction, the poetry, the spirituality do a job now. Their place in history will be judged by their success in helping to keep the community the writing serves alive, safer, together, comforted in sickness and in loss" (174). Holleran agrees: this writing will be judged "as writing published in wartime is, by its effect on the people fighting" (*Ground Zero* 17).

This idea that the appropriate measure of writing is its impact on the continued existence and well-being of the community is the valuating principle of any ethnic or national literature; it is why Isaac Bashevis Singer is important to Yiddish culture, why the slave narratives undergird all African-American writing in this country, why the underground Russian writers of the last fifty years will be treasured by generations of Russian readers. All such writing has as its innermost principle the act of bearing witness. To bear witness is to declare oneself, to declare oneself present, to declare oneself in the presence of what has come to be. This is the original discourse, the primary word, the logos that opens a space in which we can be present to one another. It is this space that allows a community to come into being, for this is the site of the action of culture and the possibility of memory. Those who bear witness carry the soul of the community, the stories of what it has done and what it has suffered, and open the possibility of its existence in memory through time and beyond death.

This understanding of writing and its inherent nature and excellence stands in opposition to all ideas of universal literary standards, the presence of which is always an outstanding characteristic of the hegemonic urge of any dominant and dominating class, group, or nation. In literary culture the assertion of universal standards of judgment is always the tip-off to the urge to dominate, to subdue the different, to draw all into a uniform order. You reach for the universal when you don't want to tolerate diversity, politically speaking, when you want to abolish the existential fact of human plurality.

This is, of course, an outstanding fact about the literary culture in America today, as anyone who has the misfortune of being in a profession that requires the reading of a large cross-section of book reviews can testify to, or as a brief glance at the furious defenses of the canon coming from our reactionary, but still dominant, cultural commentators attests to. In spite of the fact that this country is composed of a loose assortment of variegated and astonishingly numerous communities all superimposed upon one another, that virtually every individual American participates in a number of overlapping communities, each with its own culture—as a woman, say, who is also Jewish, a lesbian, and an academic—the organs of cultural definition in this country seem hell-bent on asserting a uniform and shared culture, which is in fact a myth, an obfuscation, a curtain drawn over the real mechanics of cultural creation today. The purpose, of course, is to assert control—to absorb those creations which can be assimilated to the cultural amalgam of the dominant class without upsetting the applecart, and, at the same time, to peripheralize the rest into a marginal, regional, special interest, minority reservation—colorful perhaps, worth a visit as a tourist, but in some basic way not the real thing.

This has been the root problem with the reception of works of gay writers by the mainstream press in the last decade. And it is only heightened when the writing concerns AIDS, for as long as the mainstream press does not participate in the community of crisis, which may be defined as those who choose to be affected by AIDS, as long as the mainstream press sees AIDS as something that happens to "other people," it will continue to judge this writing and these writers in terms of conventional aesthetic categories: is this aesthetically pleasing? Does it constitute an advance in the career of the writer? In short, the media will continue to miss the point.

A revealing instance can be found in the long, joint review that *Time* magazine printed in 1988 of three books provoked by the AIDS crisis: Paul Monette's *Borrowed Time,* Andrew Holleran's *Ground Zero,* and Alice Hoffman's *At Risk,* a novel by a heterosexual woman about an eleven-year-old white girl—a gymnast, no less—who got AIDS from a blood transfusion—what they call "an innocent victim." It was utterly predictable that the book that had the strongest impact on the gay community and on those affected by AIDS, Monette's *Borrowed Time,* was the book *Time* found most disagreeable. "*Borrowed Time* demands a sympathetic response instead of inviting one," complained the magazine, as if this constituted an unwonted imposition on the reader by the author (Sheppard 68–69). Would they have made the same complaint about Nedezda Mandelstam's memoirs or the tale of any Holocaust survivor, one wonders. Oddly enough, the reviewer didn't notice that the reason Holleran neither invites nor demands sympathy from straight readers is that he assumes that all his readers are gay, for this is clearly whom he is speaking to when he sits at his typewriter. Of course, the best book of the lot, according to *Time,* was Hoffman's account of an "innocent victim": "Hoffman gets the blend of hope and despair just right," approved *Time,* as if the author were whipping up a cake. What can this possibly mean? Is there a mixture of hope and despair that is just right? Is it right in all cases, or just in this instance? What precisely constitutes hope when your eleven-year-old daughter is dying of AIDS? What the reviewer really meant is that his sensibilities were not unduly disturbed, that his spirit was agitated but still soothed in a pleasing manner. If you want to see the essential vulgarity of this purely aesthetic response, just imagine someone saying, "Anne Frank got the blend of hope and despair just right."

In the gay literary community there was much heated debate about *At Risk* and a good deal of bitterness about the fact that this work of fiction far outsold any other novel on AIDS. While I believe that no author can be told what he or she can or cannot write about, this anger did not seem a surprising response. One could imagine a novel about an eleven-year-old Christian girl in Hannover who, through some mix-up one day on the street, is caught in one of the round-ups of Jews and "mistakenly" sent to Auschwitz—the "mistake" here is equivalent to "accidentally" getting AIDS. This is a perfectly legitimate subject for a novel, but if the book detailed the suffering of this child and her family while virtually ignoring the fate of the Jews at Auschwitz, one would not be surprised to get a chilly reception in the Jewish press. And if that book far outsold any other novel about the Holocaust, one would not be surprised to find bitterness in the hearts of many Jews. This is a hypothetical example, but there was in reality a similar debate over *The Confessions of Nat Turner.* All arguments aside, the point of the matter is that there *was* a heated and public debate—as there should have been—but I did not see one reviewer outside the gay press raise the issue with *At Risk,* and, in fact, few reviewers inside the gay press did either. And surely the matter was worth discussing.

In fact, it raises a serious and troubling question about the judgment of contemporary works of fiction. When I read Allen Barnett's extraordinary story "The *Times* as It Knows Us"—the title signals the sheer contempt this gay New Yorker has for our "newspaper of record" —the author's unblinking vision of the harrowing events that take place during one weekend in a not untypical gay summer house in The Pines both exhausted and impressed me. The story's power derives from its understatement, its lack of hysteria, and its unbending courage to imagine things as they are right now for many of us. It is not an unfamiliar story to me or my friends; it's one I recognize only too well, yet I found it almost unbearable to read. The fact that Barnett's imagination did not buckle under the weight of this horror steadied me and convinced me of the magnitude of his achievement. But what, I wondered, would a straight reader make of it? Would such a reader feel the unstated pressure that made it difficult for me to breathe? And, if not, was I saying that a straight friend of mine would be in no position, would have no right, to judge this story because she did not have first-hand experience of what the story was about?—a position that made me very uncomfortable. When I raised the issue with Barnett himself, he thought a moment and said, "You know, I saw a teenager, a black girl, on the subway today reading Toni Morrison's *The Bluest Eye,* a book that had an incredible impact on me. And I realized that the book could never have the meaning for me that it would have for her. And I was very glad she was reading it, for she is the audience."

For me this little story neatly raises the question of the plurality of cultures in which we live. In one of the last great works of the imperial spirit, T. E. Lawrence wrote in *The Seven Pillars of Wisdom* that to try to view reality simultaneously through the veils of two different cultures would drive a man mad. Though this sounds convincing when you come upon it in that remarkable book, one remembers that Kierkegaard and Nietzsche, the first two thinkers for whom modernity as such was a problematic issue—indeed a crisis—both characterized modernity, or perhaps the crisis hidden within it, as the ability or the necessity of holding contradictory ideas in the mind simultaneously. "Contradictory" was perhaps inexact, but the collapse of a unifying tradition that could take disparate elements and order them into a more or less uniform, or at least noncontradictory, whole, this collapse of tradition is indisputable and glaringly the fundamental datum of twentieth-century culture, articulated over and over again in the works of our thinkers, poets, and artists. By now it should be quite clear to everyone: the center did not hold. And with the collapse of the authority of tradition, all cultures, not only all present but all past cultures, regained a certain viability as a veil that one might borrow to see certain aspects of reality more clearly, as when Picasso raided African art for forms and principles that could rejuvenate his own.

The resulting situation, it seems to me—with all due respect to Lawrence of Arabia—is that today we see reality precisely through a multitude of veils simultaneously. And while this may require some fancy footwork and a greater mental and spiritual dexterity, by no means will it necessarily drive us mad.

All the questions, objections, and arguments about the existence of a separate and distinct gay culture—and the deep-seated hostility with which the spokespeople for the dominant culture in this country react to this possibility—rest on a mistaken notion of the relationship between the two. It is not, as they think, a question of the Greeks versus the barbarians, which in essence boils down to those who have culture versus those who don't, *hoi barbaroi,* the barbarians who babble, who have no language (don't speak Greek) and thus no culture. This paradigm of how a plurality of cultures coexists always comes down to a power relation, a hostile power relation: us versus them. But we *are* a them, each one of us. I am a white American gay man. I participate in gay culture, but I also participate quite actively in mainstream American culture. And, in fact, through my reading of the remarkable burst of superb writing by African-American women in the last decade and a half, not to speak of black music in general, I get to participate in black culture. And when I read Maxine Hong Kingston and Amy Tan, I get to see life in this country through the veil of Chinese-American culture.

These cultures all exist simultaneously, inexactly superimposed upon each other, a great palimpsest, creating a moiré effect in the soul that is the basic texture of cultural life today. And when groups of us—urban male Jews or African Americans or Chinese Americans or gay people—spin our veils, we are creating garments for the spirit which we can share.

Allen Barnett can share *The Bluest Eye,* though perhaps it will never have the resonance and depth for him that it will for an African-American girl. Then again, none of us can participate in Greek tragedy with the transparent clarity it must have had for contemporary Athenians. But still we read it. Which is precisely why we have Greek scholars, specialists who not only tend and preserve the work and its meaning but try to clear away the obscurity that an ever-lengthening distance between us and the work creates.

Time, of course, is not the only type of distance; there are psychic distances, between, for instance, the souls of black folk in America and the dominant American culture, between an emerging gay sensibility and straight America, between those who are living through the maelstrom of AIDS and the rest of the country. But we can bridge these distances by the active power of the imagination, that power, as Hannah Arendt used to say, that makes present that which is absent, that makes near that which is far, that power which is the root and source of all human understanding.

Those who are living through AIDS are spinning an astonishing garment for the spirit, one that offers its gift not only to those stricken but to all who care to reach, to participate in the great life of the imagination and spirit that is human culture. Gay culture is a necessity for us and an offering to the rest. At the moment, the dominant culture mainly rejects the gift and spurns the giver, which is a great foolishness.[4] The gift asks only to be taken, and in that sharing we begin to participate in the communities of all peoples. In that sharing we begin to learn how to live among a plurality of peoples and to move among a multiplicity of cultures, with whom we share the Earth even as they share with us the riches of their experiences and the wealth of their spirit.

Notes

1. The *Native's* first article ran on 18 May 1981; The Centers For Disease Control's first report in the *Morbidity And Mortality Weekly Report* ran on 5 June 1981.

2. Of course, the people I am discussing do not exhaust the list of courageous writers who have responded to the epidemic in their work; there are many more, and with time we will no doubt get more balanced overviews of the subject. I have concentrated on the works and writers I have been most involved with, through the happenstance of admiration, friendship, or professional association.

3. See, for instance, the comments of John Preston, Paul Monette, Edmund White, Andrew Holleran, and Larry Duplechan in *Tribe* 1.2 (Spring 1990): 3–29; and 1.3: 44–51.

4. See, for instance, the remarkably shallow essay by Edward Hoagland in *Esquire*, "Shhh! Our Writers Are Sleeping!" (July 1990: 57) in which he bemoans the fact that American writers of fiction avoid the major social issues of the day. Although he mentions AIDS in passing, he seems utterly unaware of the extent and depth of the literature responding to this particular issue of the day. It would seem that it is Hoagland who is asleep, especially since he also seems quite unaware of the central themes of African-American women writers in the last decade. Or perhaps the problems lies in Hoagland's understanding of the phrase "our writers."

Works Cited

Arendt, Hannah. "Epilogue: Reflections On The Hungarian Revolution." *The Origins Of Totalitarianism.* New York: Harcourt, Brace, Jovanovich, 1957.

Dawidoff, Robert. "Memorial Day, 1988." *Personal Dispatches: Writers Confront AIDS.* Ed. John Preston. New York: St. Martin's Press, 1989.

Dillard, Annie. "Write Till You Drop." *New York Times Book Review* 28 May 1989.

Foucault, Michel. *The Birth Of The Clinic.* New York: Vintage Books, 1975.

Holleran, Andrew. *Ground Zero.* New York: William Morrow, 1988.

——. "Personal Dispatches: Gay Writers And AIDS." *Tribe* 2.2 (Spring 1990).

Jack, Damien. "From the Dance to Ground Zero: An Interview with Andrew Holleran." *The New York Native* 5 December 1988.

Kaufman, David. "AIDS: The Cultural Response." *Horizon Magazine* 30.9 (November 1987).

Kramer, Larry. *Reports from the holocaust.* New York: St. Martin's Press, 1989.

Lassell, Michael. "How to Watch Your Brother Die." *Gay And Lesbian Poetry In Our Time.* Ed. Morse and Larkin. New York: St. Martin's Press, 1988.

Monette, Paul. *Afterlife.* New York: Crown, 1990.

——. *Half Way Home.* New York: Crown, 1991.

——. *Love Alone.* New York: St. Martin's Press, 1989.

O'Conner, Michael. "Interview With Victor Bumbalo." *Mandate* (January 1990).

Pettit, Sarah. "Bearing Witness: An Interview With John Preston." *Outweek* 25 (10 December 1990).

Preston, John. "AIDS Writing: Comments Made at the 1990 Outwrite Conference, San Francisco." Unpublished manuscript.

——. "An Essay." *Tribe* 1.2 (Spring 1990).

Sheppard, R. Z. "Journals of the Plague Years." *Time* 18 July 1988.

Shilts, Randy. "Talking AIDS To Death." *Esquire* March 1989.

Stomberg, Mark. "Deleriously Unique: An Interview With Paul Monette" *The New York Native* 26 March 1990.

White, Edmund. "Palace Days." *The Darker Proof: Stories From A Crisis.* New York: New American Library, 1988.

■ LARRY EBMEIER

Requiem Evita

There are birds in my chimney. When it was bitter cold outside, they chirped and fluttered and flapped about, sounding as though the Boston Strangler got hold of their throats. Do birds have throats? Of a sort, I suppose they do. It was windy that day, and as gusts swept the chimney ports way up there somewhere, it sounded almost like low, distant, steady thunder, thunder like an approaching storm on the plains of my youth. It sounded like thunder when everything else in the house—that is to say, the furnace, refrigerator, toilet, water softener, and electric heater—was all shut off. And through this low, distant thunder, these birds twittered away. Presently, some of them sounded as though they'd gotten inside the chimney and landed on top of the damper.

And I thought, Well, what if they're little bird offspring who've fallen out of the nest higher up in the chimney and are trapped down here atop the damper cover? If I open that damper, they'll spill right onto the hearth, which is empty and hard and barren, as I rarely use my fireplace. And there they'll be, right inside my house, tiny flesh-colored bird offspring. That's how bird offspring look when they're especially young, before feathering: small, bloated, flesh-colored, vein-infested things with oversize eyes, undersize beaks, and wrinkles up the backs of their wobbly little heads (wrinkles reminiscent of their elderly or sickly human counterparts). There they'll be, flapping and flailing away like beached fish on my clean, barren, unused hearth, screeching at me to "Do something, for God's sake!"

And do they expect me to get bundled up, go to the basement, dig out the ladder (a heavy, thirty-foot metal extension ladder), put it up in horribly negative wind chill, and risk life and limb in a foolish, bleeding-hearted attempt to restore them to their nest way up there somewhere, a nest I cannot be certain I could even find inside that tall, mysterious, dark chimney, a nest perhaps already abandoned by their mother bird? Is that what these tiny, flailing, screeching, flesh-colored bird offspring now expect?

I read somewhere that once you handle bird offspring, even to return them to their nest, their bird mothers abandon them. That doesn't make sense, of course, so it's probably true, since nature is, I know, cruel, messy, and, most of all, illogical. And even if their parents didn't fly off, the bird offspring would probably just fall out of that nest again, perhaps an hour or two later, the way a helpless but spiteful infant will keep dropping a spoon from the highchair, no matter how many times you retrieve it. And there I'd be, back in my living room, listening to distant thunder mingled with the sounds of fallen bird offspring, those pesky birds in my chimney that make me think of AIDS.

Nature has never made much sense to me, even though I grew up on a farm in south central Nebraska. In fact, I used to imagine myself "at war with nature," and grew quite fond of flinging that phrase back at my relatives whenever they put to me the inevitable question: "Do you want to farm your dad's place?"

"No," I would smile curtly. "That will be quite impossible, as I am at war with nature."

It became quite a joke, nature and me. I told my friends that I didn't dare eat anything unless it was full of preservatives. "Fresh fruit, vegetables, and milk will kill you," I warned. And the weather, I could always easily prove, did cruel things to me. My flowers always fizzled, potted palms inevitably perished, and there was my lawn, laced with yellows and browns.

But when AIDS happened, the concept of being "at war with nature" grew far less funny than it once seemed.

Confronting AIDS as a monolith is dizzying, overwhelming, and humanly impossible, but individual to individual, the noises and news, whether bad or good, give me glimpses of myself.

"It isn't because they're afraid of catching it, but I think they just can't or don't want to deal with the end of existence, which, in my case, is a speeded-up mirror image of their own," explains my friend Dwight in steady, quiet tones. He is talking about his biggest disappointment since becoming AIDS-symptomatic: the way so many of his friends have quietly disappeared. Dwight's gentle eyes seem to have grown larger, moister, and deeper as his body has thinned. It's as if the part of his vitality that disappeared from his limbs and trunk took refuge in his eyes.

"Just because you know your days are (more tightly) numbered doesn't mean you should stop and give up or suddenly try to jam a year into every day. Both are pretty much impossible. So you might change a few things, maybe do some things you'd otherwise put off, but mostly what you have to do is go on living from day to day pretty much the way you always have. I don't really see how anyone can expect much else, do you?" There's a lot of American Great Plains survivalist common sense in Dwight.

Beyond the dizzying death counts, the explosions of anger, fear, and sorrow, beyond post–Rock Hudson–inspired star-studded mega-benefits, big rallies, and The Quilt, it has settled into a protracted, quiet struggle—a series of private battles, pathetic and courageous, commonsensical and haphazard, bitter and lonely—tragic togetherness. Not unlike cancer, it's become one more too-soon way to die; no worse, no better, not necessarily redeeming, not always heroic, not even a fad any longer.

Thursday morning came after more sleep than usual. It came gray, cold, and dreary. Like me, Thursday morning was having a bitch of a time waking up. Thursday morning came pointless and relentless, like unwanted conversation at the long end of a less than enjoyable party, when I'm tired and drunk.

I am staring at the oily, pitching surface of dark brown coffee catching incandescent light from the spot above. It slams my head into a strobelike disco gear, then half-hypnotizes it, so that I must steady myself with both hands on the countertop.

The house is a mess; not a wreck, but, like me, a situation reflecting recent absence and neglect, a slippage in control. This used to upset me, but lately, when I find myself seeing it, I feel more wonder and less regret at these bits of litter accumulating in my wake.

The mail arrives earlier than usual, before eleven. Retrieving it, wet, curled-up October leaves are mashed into rainwatered terrazzo beneath my rubber thong sandals, forming a slippery, syrupy seal. I try in vain to shake the leaves free, only to step in more, so I shake my fist at the golden canopy of the great linden tree filtering and amplifying wet, gray light into something unusual, bright, seemingly artificial, as though this were the planet Krypton and I was shaking my fist at its red sun.

Not much mail here. "Mine," I mutter, sorting it by dropping it into sloppy piles on carpeted stairs in the hallway. "Mine, Don, Don, garbage, garbage, Don, garbage, mine."

The church bulletin announces David's death.

I am still far too sleepy and disoriented to believe it is the David I fear it could be. Probably lots of Davids in the church, I say to myself. Lots of Davids in the world, period. But the way everything else has gone this week, I decide it probably is who I fear it is, and I know that David's death is just one more piece of my own miserable luck rather than his.

Still, it will take me a day of denial and Don's official verification to confirm it. Don's official verification comes the following evening in the form of a torn-out section of the Sunday newspaper obituary lying like a sunbather across the top of my electric blue electric typewriter. At the very top in the left-hand corner of the page is a summary list of names of today's deceased, so that one doesn't have to scan through a whole column of stories that might not contain the dead person one is seeking. Just thumb down this handy upper left-hand corner alphabetized list, and if he's not there, try again tomorrow. David is there all right. The very first name. Right at the top.

Don, my lover and also a friend of David, has placed this obituary section here, knowing that if it sunbathes across the top of my typewriter I cannot possibly miss this very important, very official piece of bad news. Don has long since proven his efficiency at relaying bad news in impossible-to-miss ways, officially, bureaucratically, like an administrative secretary. I appreciate Don's preciseness, but really, I'd have preferred he just tell me, rather than convey David's death in the format of executive memo and report. The sunbathing piece of newspaper says, "Died Saturday, 9-30-89."

"This last September Saturday, this day full of lazy heat and languid fall sunshine spent enjoying a drive around Kansas City having golden philosophical conversation with a kindred spirit of the closest rank." That's how I recorded the day in my journal. How was I to know David was dying at the very same time? I wonder if he'd be glad to know how much I enjoyed his last day on earth?

"Wouldn't it be nice," I said to Greg, as we puttered around Kansas City in his tiny blue Tercel on David's last day on Earth, "if I hadn't been born out here on the plains to strict Catholic parents during the dark ages when our kind had hardly a classification, much less a justification? Wouldn't it be nice if I'd been, as the song goes, 'Born Free,' free to come out young, like they do today in a big city, to liberal, encouraging parents, surrounded by admiring peers and helpful role models?"

Greg knew someone like that. His name was Chris. His parents were Unitarians. He came out at sixteen. He was young, handsome, and now lives in the Bay area. Now in his early thirties, he's also been diagnosed HIV-positive.

When I was sixteen I was at my ugliest and least youthful. I was fat, cautious, controlled, and suspicious during those years when most members of my species are at their most beautiful, athletic, carefree, and innocent. Those tender, young, pretty years we call youth, I stifled in passage during the dark ages. It was a different time.

"We were lucky," said Greg that afternoon during that philosophical, puttering drive around Kansas City, "to be so closeted so long—just long enough, as it turned out, that we didn't fall prey to the dreaded Plague."

David had receded in recent years to just an acquaintance, a dim memory of someone I used to know and fully expected to exist as a patch of human terrain upon my psychological landscape. His was never a life I fully understood, approved of, or tried to emulate. His chief claim to local fame was that he made a very elegant, tall, somewhat ephemerally convincing drag queen and, for his age, had uncommonly smooth skin.

Most vividly, I recall the excitement, grandeur, and warmth surrounding a segment of my own coming out in an early 1980s summer show he did at the old Hollywood Bar in Omaha. All I did was videotape the show, but it was a day spent with David and his gay friends (a new experience for me), a day spent drink-ing, dancing, and partying, then driving home alone in my big white convertible, driving beneath stars through warm August air that felt as friendly in the middle of the night as amniotic fluid. How could I help but reflect upon how wonderful it all was to be alive.

David's nervous hands once trimmed my hair. I could smell ciga-rettes on his breath, while I sat so smugly still, wondering if he found me attractive. I still own a collection of programs and brochures from "Hellfire XI," a B&D/S&M woodsie he found southwest of Grand Rapids, Michigan. What excitement flamed in his eyes as he spoke of Tops and Bottoms, Dungeon Masters, and the Hades Clearing. I felt somewhat ashamed at only dimly comprehending and instinctively recoiling from what he clearly found to be a "garden of delights." Is it wrong, or even relevant now, to feel embarrassed over being so green, so ignorant then, even at age thirty-two?

David's death, regardless of the official newspaper date, came that dreary Thursday morning to me, even though he died the Saturday before, because at least half of each death's significance is its realiza-tion by those of us left living.

Confronting AIDS as a monolith is humanly impossible, but individual to individual, the noises and news, whether bad or good, give us glimpses of ourselves. We are hardened by anger, misunderstanding, and fear, softened and lifted by love and courage that comes almost magically from out of nowhere. Our singularlity and aloneness are shattered like a black, newly formed lava shell from an erupting volcano, a black shell riding over red, searing, molten masses, flowing and coursing in torrents beneath, black giving way to let the molten lava burst forth in a new, bright-red finger of fire forming yet another channel in tune with mass and gravity, until it too slows, blackens hard, and is stopped.

Ultimately, some of the lava fingers reach the sea, dipping their red, hot ends into breaking waves amidst a fanfare of steam and thunderous explosion.

Within and without the community, as within and without each individual, there is this painful, fiery process of reality and reconciliation, like volcanic lava seeking the sea. Through our friends, enemies, lovers, and strangers our fiery rivers flow, changing channels constantly, until finally, reaching some acceptance, some end, like the seawater, cooling and coming to rest in a fanfare of bursting steam and cleansing foam.

Rising early that chilly Wednesday October morning with Paul and Bryan seemed like a downright dumb idea at the time. It was the last morning of my long Twin Cities weekend, a weekend spent gathering "Minneapolis Facts" for a book I had in progress, but also a weekend spent exposing myself to old friends and new strangers. There had been a fifty-hour AIDS prayer vigil, after which I'd met Bryan, a thin, reddish-blond man, made to seem all the more frail because of his height. Bryan had been introduced by Paul, a dark-eyed, black-haired, wiry, young Italian who was my host for the weekend. Paul had branded Bryan "Really, just a screamer, Larry," then proved it by demonstrating how well the two of them could squeal, dish, and dismiss away the hours, until I felt as awkward and out of place as I had when I'd used the wrong restroom at Little Amana.

That cold morning, as Bryan drove Paul to the Amtrak station over in Saint Paul, they shrieked, giggled, gossiped, and blocked all the heater vents, while I huddled, shivering with a sense of resignation and irrelevance in the back seat of Bryan's cheap, battered little Chevrolet, wishing I'd slept in until some sane hour, risen leisurely, and taken coffee at that cozy little Greek café in the "uptown" area.

Excitedly, Paul and Bryan "argued" over the best mode of transpor-

tation to Washington, where they were both going to participate in
the great AIDS march and Names Project. "Paul, honey," cooed
Bryan like Mae West, "this girl isn't messing around spending thirty-
two hours on some old train like youuu are. She's flying!"

"Well, maybe Miss Thing should see what she *could* find to mess
around with for thirty-two hours on the train. I've ridden the rails all
my life, sweetie, and I do mean *ridden!*"

It was still dark, as we sped east on I-94 jammed full of taillights
darting about in front of us like nervous insects. I could only wonder
what on earth Bryan and I would talk about on the return trip from
the station, after we dropped off Paul, for I hardly knew Bryan and
certainly couldn't "dish" on his level—or any other level, for that
matter. It would be a silent, awkward drive back, him smoking his
cigarettes that PWAs aren't supposed to, and me staring out my
window, feeling like a Methodist trapped in a Catholic church, inca-
pable of following Mass.

I liked Bryan, what little I knew of him, but I was also frightened
of him, frightened of the tears I'd seen from him at the prayer vigil,
frightened of how much more he seemed to know and to have seen of
life and the world than I, frightened of the way he chain-smoked
those cigarettes, when he had a debilitating terminal illness to battle,
and, most of all, frightened by the fact that I'd just finished writing a
novel about his disease.

What could he tell me, if he told me anything, about AIDS? What
would he tell me that I'd curse myself for missing or having gotten
wrong in my book, now that it was too late? And should I give him an
autographed copy? Or would that simply depress, or worse, infuriate
him? Here was a tailor-made parcel of my audience, a real person
with the disease. I should be thrilled and proud of my work, literally
chomping at the bit to have him read it.

But instead of chomping, I was chattering—with chilly irrelevance
and fear, the same kind of fear that had washed over me months
earlier on a beautiful early April Sunday afternoon in Des Moines.
There I sat among an elegant audience enjoying brunch in an old
mansion, while the actor Michael Kearnes gave a speech on behalf of
his group, ACA, Artists Confronting AIDS. The speech closed out
four days of AIDS-awareness activities in the Iowa capital, activities
ranging from plays to movies to a concert by the Twin Cities Men's
Chorus, of which Paul, incidentally, was a member.

Through Kearnes's speech, which told of his overcoming "self-
loathing" by finding a "cause" in AIDS, I gazed about the big hall
furnished in stately antiques, sun streaming in through big French

windows and a breathtaking leaded glass skylight, and, amidst gallons of fresh tulips, daisies, and carnations, from behind flowered china and white linen, tried to keep my mind off the fact that here was my audience. These people, or at least some of them, would soon read my first novel about AIDS. Would it be good enough? Did I even have the right to create it? How could I presume to know more, or feel more, than all these people did? I wasn't a victim and, so far, no one I knew closely, no one I loved, had it. Lincoln, Nebraska, wasn't exactly the epicenter of the epidemic. In fact, many in our regional Midwest community seemed blissfully ignorant of "safe sex." So how dare I romanticize or embellish such horrible reality from such a distance?

Exploring the beauty gathered in that grand room that morning, it struck me how common it had suddenly become for a gay man, for me, to confront the spectre of mass sickness and sudden death, be it my own, that of a friend, or of those I had only heard about. It's a spectre I could not possibly have imagined just a decade earlier, struggling to come out, or even three years before, when I'd undertaken to write *Tweeds.* "Confront AIDS?" Corey Reese, the novel's hero might have whined incredulously. "Why, I don't even know how to ask a man out on a date, and you're asking me to confront a fatal disease?"

Kearnes's speech was full of words like *feeling, giving, sharing, powerful, loving, healthy,* and *alive*—too full for my comfort. It seemed brimful of gushing emotion that had pervaded the gay community as surely as the death that had spawned it, emotion cast about too freely, too joyfully before grim, silent reality set in.

In Paul Theroux's *Old Patagonian Express: By Train through the Americas,* mention is made about the overemphasis on pain and suffering of saints, martyrs, and Jesus in the religious artwork of Latin America. So many rituals, frescoes, paintings, and statues seem too gory, too bloody, as if they are bizarre indulgences, almost celebrations of physical torture and excruciating suffering. But Theroux postulates that this is probably because the natives' concept of religious heroes' sufferings must somehow outdo their own, which is considerable in lands wracked by everyday horrific poverty, starvation, disease, and death.

I became suddenly afraid, that beautiful, sunny April morning in 1987, that perhaps I had messed in some inadequate way with a community subject too full of pain, sorrow, and emotion. I was privately afraid of the same thing that chilly morning in October, freeze-shiver-hunched in the rear seat of Bryan's cold, clattering

Chevy, as he and Paul rushed to embrace that grand Washington outpouring of emotion while dishing hilariously back and forth in high style.

Suddenly, I heard a mournful trumpet fanfare, then a choir of voices in atonal unison: "Requiem Evita! Requiem Evita!" Bryan had inserted his tape cassette soundtrack of the musical *Evita*. A man began to sing a critique on the funeral of Eva Peron. He sang about what a circus Buenos Aires had become in her wake, but at the same time he conceded that this was certainly the way to go, if you had to go, a grand funeral like Eva Peron's.

Bryan settled back comfortably in his seat, left hand gripping the wheel, right hand on the gearshift, and began to sing along, loudly, happily, as if the song were an old friend he'd just met at his favorite bar. He grinned proudly, defiantly into the first glimpses of morning light breaking to the east over that dark, chaotic sea of traffic. He gave Paul's leg a slap and sang louder. He sang about Eva Peron's style; he sang about how she was the "best show in town." He sang along with the man on the tape, who wondered how Argentina would survive without her.

To me, this just made everything all the more absurd. Now, instead of dishing and shrieking, queenish Bryan was belting out the soundtrack to *Evita*, serenading Paul, who laughed along good-naturedly, but clearly looked as if he'd rather Bryan shut up. His look only sparked Bryan to greater heights. He flipped the volume higher, until the music came distorted and crackling through the small, inexpensive speakers in his battered, tiny car sandwiched between hurtling, killer traffic rushing east on I-94—and sang louder.

Then, all at once it made some cosmic kind of sense. Here was a man who'd led his own circus of a life and now faced a premature end, an abbreviated existence by most standards, just like Eva Peron, who was cut down in the flower of life. To Bryan, a funeral like Eva Peron's, even if only in his imagination sparked by a modern musical, seemed the perfect gigantic ending. The fantasy lifted his spirit, reassured him, made him proud of what he was and glad for what had been. "How will they live without her?" he laughed and sang on. "What will they do without her?"

Paul was much too caught up in the elation of his morning, anticipating his train trip to Washington. "Please, dear," he playfully chastised Bryan, "don't play that silly old song again! For God's sake, turn that awful thing down, before your car blows up!"

And Bryan certainly wasn't singing to me, yet I'd heard him, loud and clear. I knew now that he and I would indeed have something to talk about on the long drive back to Minneapolis, and maybe, as someone "messing around" with the chronicling of painful, emotional, even horrifying times, I wasn't exactly missing everything. It was a fine thing to witness, Bryan's flamboyant courage and good humor in the face of his plight. To have seen it and sort of understood, or even cared, made me feel close to him, myself, and especially my craft.

Writing about AIDS
for Young Adults

In 1985, a twenty-two-year-old neighbor died of something then called GRIDS, or Gay Related Immune Deficiency Syndrome. I had watched for two years while this young man grew thinner as rumors about him spread in the community. A bad joke went around: There's good news and there's bad news. The bad news is I'm homosexual. The good news is I'm dying.

When Bud was going to high school here, there was nothing to indicate he was any different from the other boys. He was popular and versatile, a good student, a very good basketball player, a fellow who always had a date at the school dances and summer beach parties. He had a younger sister who adored him, and when he went to New York University to study filmmaking, it was always an event for her when he came home, dragging college buddies with him. Bud was not a loner. He was always part of a group.

Bud came home reluctantly in 1983—reluctantly because coming home meant coming out to his parents and his sister . . . and ultimately to the community. There seemed no place else for him to go to die. No one knew a lot about this illness, but enough was known for people to be fearful and rejecting.

A catering service refused to do the annual Christmas party at the family's home that year. A practical nurse would not sign on for duty there. Friends who used to drop in frequently and casually stayed away. People whispered that Bud had gay cancer . . . that it was lethal . . . that it could be caught from dishes, linens, a handshake, breathing in the same air he breathed out.

Late in 1984 I began to think of writing a novel about this, and I actually began it a few days before the new year. I had decided to tell the story of a young boy and his older brother, and in the mysterious way the mind works as it gears up for a project, I got a clear image of a kite flying at night, small battery lights illuminating it. I saw a teenage boy with his very young brother down on a beach, explaining differences in people by using the kite.

"Yes, most kites go up in the daytime . . . but some kites go up at night."

"Aren't they afraid of the dark?" the small boy somewhere in my head asked.

"No, they're different from day kites. They go up alone, on their own, and they're not afraid to be different."

So began the mental dialogue that so often precedes the actual writing . . . and I began to think of who the other characters would be and what their parents would be like. One thing I knew for certain: this novel, unlike any other, would need some extra-interesting trappings, for if there are two subjects teens don't warm to, one is homosexuality and the other is illness.

I am a great fan of rock music. I rarely write about it because it dates a book, the groups and musicians coming and going so quickly. Where I live there are a lot of rock stars in residence, and I've interviewed some and read other local writers' interviews of them.

I was convinced that in this book I could use some of my material because surely this was a disease that would not be around for long either, and even so would change, would not be at all the same in five or ten years, thus outdating my fiction. And wasn't this the perfect book, too, for a discussion of rock stars and rock music? For surely they were night kites, most of them; yesterday's losers, so many of them; people who did not walk in step, and never had. It is all through their music.

I began to invent Nicki, the girlfriend of my younger brother's best pal, a girl who patterns herself after Madonna, who wears funky clothes and loves rock music and collects stories of the stars she sees on MTV. An outsider who doesn't fit in with the others. A night kite.

I began to write.

Then I began to grind my teeth at night . . . and to fear as time went on that with *Night Kites,* I was committing professional suicide. How would teachers answer the questions this illness provoked? Not just questions about "normal" sex, but about homosexuality? What would parents say? Wasn't I asking for trouble with a book on this subject?

Still, I couldn't get the story out of my head, and as time went on, I began to realize what was happening was very important, too: a much larger issue than I'd ever dreamed.

The name of the illness was changed from GRIDS to AIDS, and I began to read more and more about it.

In early 1986 when I finished the book, I was still apprehensive, even worried that my publisher might not want my book at all, that the subject was too hot to handle. And I began to wonder if I should have written about a child who had gotten AIDS through a blood transfusion . . . some safer presentation . . . some greater distancing so that readers would be more sympathetic and not so ready to vent their fears and anxieties about homosexuality.

But Harper & Row accepted the book immediately, with only minor changes, none having to do with the subject matter, and Night Kites became the first young adult book about AIDS.

Sometimes when I visited schools after it was first published, I was asked not to speak about it: any book but the one dealing with AIDS. Eventually, though, that attitude disappeared. AIDS had been mainstreamed by the time the paperback came out in 1987. Now, instead of being asked not to discuss it, letters were arriving from teachers wondering, for instance, why I didn't caution the young people in the book to use condoms! Condoms were a regular part of classroom discussion in most schools by then! Had anyone forecast that when I was beginning the book, I would have insisted there was no possibility, ever, of that!

A Ryan White still brings out the celebrities to publically mourn the death of someone from AIDS. Never mind the many, many homosexual men who have made this world a better, brighter place by what they painted, or wrote, or designed, or interpreted or portrayed and who died from AIDS. We still feel safer saluting a child with a blood disorder than allying ourselves in any way with addiction or "abnormality." But the illness has forced some compassion on every community, even the most reluctant.

In 1990 on Long Island, I went to train to be a buddy to an AIDS patient, helping him or her with daily chores and being there as a friend. So many volunteers showed up that we had to split into two groups: a very good sign. At the Long Island high schools where I speak a lot, I sense the kids' rejection of drugs, the new scornful attitude toward users, when not too long ago doing drugs was considered cool.

I know the other side of the coin, too: the growing hostility toward homosexuals, forcing many back into the shadows of lies and hiding, the way Bud lived until his last painful years.

Night Kites is still in print. I wish I could end by saying there wasn't a need for it anymore, that it was from back in time when there wasn't a cure.

Crying "Wolf!": The Genesis of an AIDS Disaster Epic

To Write or Not to Write

The idea for *A Cry in the Desert* developed in the first half of 1982. The resolve to write it grew through the remainder of that year in direct proportion to my accumulating anger and frustration.

It began with the death of an acquaintance. Strangely enough, AIDS was the motive, not the cause. A friend's lover was leaving a Las Vegas gay bar early in the morning when a group of young people in a car drove through the parking lot yelling obscenities and accusations. Gay bashing had not been common in Vegas, so apparently the young man hadn't worried about leaving the bar alone. The parking lot was sparsely lighted, and the kids in the car pulled into the shadows, where they turned out their lights and continued to call him "faggot" and "death spreader." He tried to ignore them and get out of there quickly, but they were between him and his car. As he crossed the dark, open space between rows of cars, the driver gunned his motor. The car lurched forward with tires squealing and ran over the young man, leaving him smashed and dying. There was a witness, a man sitting in his car, but he refused to get involved, claiming that he couldn't see faces or even a license number. The young man died before the ambulance got there, Vegas's first—but unrecognized—victim of AIDS. Although I heard about his death almost immediately, its true meaning wasn't made clear to me until weeks later.

At that time, my lover and I belonged to a local gay group that was supposedly devoted to consciousness raising and political activism but was primarily a social club. At one of our winter meetings, when it was too cold for a real party, we had a guest speaker, our local gay physician, who introduced us to what was then called the "Gay Plague." Little was known about it other than that it was fatal in all known cases and apparently spread through sexual contact. We listened in horror, at first in fear of our own lives, then in realization of our vulnerability beyond the disease itself. The doctor's grim warning created in me a virtual explosion of potentialities, none of them positive.

Legionnaire's disease and toxic shock syndrome had appeared in the recent past, and the concern for "innocent victims" had caused a flurry of activity among government and medical personnel as well as special interest groups. Money had been immediately appropriated, and the soothing social blanket of "We're doing all we can—we'll take care of you" was thrown over the panicked country by a sympathetic media. Here was the opportunity for us to observe society's commitment to its gay population. Even after the unsettling ERA push by women, even after the distancing of veterans from public sympathy following the Vietnam debacle, women and veterans had been embraced when a life-threatening situation developed. After all, they were family. We, too, had demanded and grudgingly received a measure of recognition and protection during the 1970s. Had we finally become mainstream, a recognized part of the social family? Would the sympathy, assurances, and money be granted to us?

The answers were predictable and discouraging. Despite warnings from the Centers for Disease Control, most levels of government refused even to acknowledge the problem. It seemed that if they admitted a health crisis existed, they would also have to admit that gays themselves existed—and in large numbers. The latter was not politically (or, to them, ethically or morally) expedient. Therefore, they refused to acknowledge the crisis. Once more, hatred and bigotry outweighed reason and even common sense. There is a curious twist to this denial, almost as if those involved denied our humanity in more than a socially metaphorical sense. It was a throwback to the pseudoscientific jargon that produced the "master race" and "pure Aryan" idiocies of the Nazi period. If gays weren't really human, then the health threat to nongays was inconsiderable. And, by extension, if only gays were infected and dying, silence on the part of those in power could serve several purposes: (1) avoid responsibility and cost indefinitely; (2) avoid political repercussions among gay-haters; (3) get rid of some, if not all, of the members of a problematic subculture. (As the years have passed, this attitude has been reinforced by the emergence of drug addicts and prostitutes as affected populations.)

Media coverage, what there was of it, was flavored more with assumptions and prejudices than with facts, thus reinforcing gay stereotypes. And to the already rampant distrust and loathing of gays was added the element of fear, which, as time passed, escalated in many to unreasonable terror. Leaders of various churches, primarily those of the fundamentalist stamp, fanned the flames of fear and loathing by pronouncing AIDS to be the just punishment of God upon gays. And they warned straights that if the disease spread to them, it was their own fault for allowing gays a place among them.

As a sometime social studies teacher and avid student of the period preceding and including World War II, I began to see disturbing parallels between the Holocaust and the current AIDS situation. In the summer of 1982, I took a course at the University of Nevada at Las Vegas devoted entirely to the Holocaust. During those weeks, I found that my perceptions were not unique. Many others I talked to had made similar links; however, no one seemed to believe the conclusions they reached. Most said, rather too quickly, "It could never happen here," and dismissed the idea. I couldn't. I decided to explore the "what if?" by creating a fictional account of the health crisis transformed into a sociopathological nightmare. Was it possible? And if possible, could I make it believable? If it were possible, even to a limited extent, I wanted to help the gay community awaken to its danger.

As a teacher, I gave more than lip service to the value of education as a preventative of social evils, and in my opinion, fiction is often a better teacher than fact, which is always limited and most often distorted. There would be many books written on AIDS in the following years, I thought, nonfiction works presenting the newly discovered medical facts, activist books berating the already obvious lethargy and apathy of government. There would be a plethora of self-help books and tragic personal accounts, both fact and fiction. I had to speak out, but none of these voices was appropriate for me. I hesitated. I would be called a scare-monger, a reactionary, an opportunist, and any number of other unflattering terms. Would I be someone crying "Wolf!" or would I be a voice crying in the wilderness? Would I be heeded to the extent that gay organizations, even a few, like the one to which I belonged in Las Vegas, would begin demanding their full rights as citizens, not only in relation to the disease, but also the security and protection of their position as human beings in a civilized modern state? Maybe they would listen; maybe not.

Prior to World War II, Japanese leaders referred to the United States as a "sleeping giant." Its apathy was hard to shake, its anger slow to rise. That same apathy (or easygoing disinterestedness, if you prefer) had in some cases been an asset. It kept us from precipitous involvement in the affairs of other nations. However, in some instances—World War II and its preceding decade, for example—that same apathy had the potential to destroy the nation. The gay community, in spite of possible disclaimers by homophobes, was (and, in general, still is) as easygoing and apathetic as the country at large. With this new crisis, fear of discovery, of death, and of retribution were being added to apathy, and the combination could be as devastating to our community as inaction was to the Jews during the Holocaust. I do not presume to understand the apparent complaisance of many Jews in their own destruction. It is one of the great mysteries in the world to me, despite all I have read on the subject. Still, I didn't want even a few gays to be destroyed by our own acquiescence. Enough of us were dying already, and many, many more would follow.

If I could visualize for our community the ultimate effects of a situation like this gotten out of hand, maybe we could make enough noise so that those who would use the situation to destroy us would have to think twice. (And here I had no qualms: there have always been those who would destroy us. They, more often than not, are the most vociferous of all. Their very excess tends to deny them credibility, but we shouldn't forget Hitler and Goebbels. They, too, were called noisy clowns, hyperbole taken to its most ridiculous.) The rattlesnake can be killed as easily as a garter snake, but its warning gives the attacker pause. I would make a noise. And if they laughed, I would at least have gotten their attention, perhaps at a critical moment. I could afford to look ridiculous. But was what I was proposing really so ridiculous? I hesitated. I wrote some and hesitated some more. Then events began to occur that gave me new impetus.

I wrote about nurses refusing to treat AIDS patients. I fantasized about discussions of quarantine on a mass scale and about morticians refusing AIDS corpses. In my fiction, hospitals refused entry of patients, insurance companies and health agencies refused payments and assistance, families turned out children, lovers turned out lovers, churches condemned from the pulpit and on national TV. Quacks plotted to fleece the unwary, and homophobes used every means at their command to turn public opinion toward the violent. Little old blue-haired ladies refused to let their hairdressers touch them. Gay waiters and chefs were fired. Witch hunts and mandatory testing were inaugurated. Gay bashings and gay deaths proliferated. Entire cities passed anti-AIDS, antigay legislation.

As I wrote, I would find the incidents I described parroted in the back pages of newspapers and magazines. What I was writing was not fiction but short-term prophecy, and the time between the writing and the actualization was shrinking. It was impossible, but it was happening. Not in one place, as in my microcosm, but in patches throughout the country and the world. How long would it be before the incidence shifted from the sporadic to the norm, and from the norm to total justification? I kept writing. Still, deep within me, I didn't want to believe what I was saying. And yet I did believe. What I couldn't foresee but only hope for was that the ultimate, violent ends I put into words would never become reality. It had to stop far short of that. Somewhere, sometime soon, reason would prevail.

Throughout our history, we Americans have committed crimes against ourselves and others through selective myopia, tunnel vision, and willful blindness. We tend to assess social situations more on hope or optimism or comfortable lies and misrepresentations than on facts or even hypotheses based on observation and past experience. A good example would be the deep-seated belief in the myth that America is a land where all people are treated equally under the law. Actuality and the overlying hype (mostly well intentioned) are so disparate as to be ludicrous. Ask a member of any minority, racial or otherwise. The correlation between American selective sight and that of Germans in the 1930s and 1940s is striking. The motives behind such actions (or inaction, as the case may be) and the morality or immorality of their results can be argued endlessly. In the final analysis, it seems to me, the results are the same. They vary in degree but not in any measure of rightness or wrongness.

It can be argued that selective sight is a universal human failing. I don't presume to disagree; on the contrary, I consider it a major sociological tenet. But making a direct parallel to Americans of the 1980s and Germans of the 1930s and 1940s brings out a violent reaction in people, a bizarre emotional admixture of self-righteousness, affront, hubris, hypocrisy, guilt, and denial. The Germans in power killed millions, as have other governments past and present. Those not in power share the guilt (again, to an arguable degree). Perhaps being equated with the German populace of that time hits such a sore spot because of the sheer magnitude of the Holocaust. Nothing in American history could possibly compare. Or could it? What of the displacement and murder of untold numbers of African Americans and Native Americans? Is there a difference between working people to death in a slave camp or on a plantation or slowly starving them to death on a reservation? Is there a difference between concentration camps and American slavery? Is there a difference between killing people with poison gas because they are Jews or communists or homosexuals, and killing by Winchester rifle or napalm or atom bomb (for economic or moral reasons)? Leaving aside all considerations of conduct during war—as war is often used as an excuse for reaching the same ends unattainable in peacetime—is there any difference between murdering eleven million people and lynching one? Finally, is there any difference between standing by and watching (that is, giving tacit consent) while someone is lynched, and making no effort to save a person dying of AIDS? I submit that there is no difference in any of the above. Degree be damned. If, as a society, we tolerate or encourage murder on any level, for any reason, we are capable of genocide. Numbers become a factor of other considerations: opportunity, motive, and elements of gain versus risk and censure.

There are those who say that nowadays we are more civilized, more enlightened. I seriously doubt it. The argument loses force when we remember that it was used by the Germans during the Holocaust to explain away rumors. It is still being used by those who deny that the Holocaust ever took place. Quite the reverse has been shown to be true: it takes an advanced technological society (we often mistake technology for civilization) to fully exploit the potential for meting out cruelty and death.

There is a corollary to the selective sight phenomenon—I think of it as the Insulation Corollary. Humans live by the death of other organisms, plant and animal. This brutal, if natural, fact is softened and even entirely removed from daily life by technology and job specialization. The man munching a hamburger gives no thought to the death of the cow. He may think that he could never slit the throat of a fellow creature himself. He is insulated from the act and the disturbing surrounding circumstances. He gives no thought to his personal responsibility and liability in the whole process of slaughter. His personal values and beliefs are rarely, if ever, brought into question due to sheer distance from the act, processing steps between the act and what he sees, and the consciously applied softening effects of advertising and packaging. Indeed, he may reject the very idea that he could be held responsible. He is insulated, not blameless (if, for argument's sake, we tie morality to killing in order to live, which is, admittedly, unfair). If confronted, he might plead all sorts of extenuating circumstances, but the hard reality is that the killing goes on, and that he is responsible (as are all of us).

One might assume that if the hamburger-eater were required to kill his own beef, his "civilized" sensibilities would be offended, and the slaughter would cease. I think this unlikely. And in our society, such a requirement would be thought ridiculous. We insist on those intermediaries who deal with unpleasantness, and any liabilities are de facto laid upon the intermediary as part of the price of employment. Thus, the SS men who gassed Jews are responsible, even though the mandate came from power figures and, ultimately, from the society at large. Should the "need" for "disposal" of undesirables be assessed here and now, we would delegate the task (along with the liability) to professionals and require that we be as little inconvenienced as possible with the unpleasant details. All that is truly needed is to (1) define a need or desire in terms acceptable to the majority; (2) strip away the humanity of the victims to make the action more compatible with outward forms; and (3) assign someone to quietly do the dirty work.

Given our history and the premise stated above, the mythical American immunity to acts of gross immorality ("It could never happen here!") disappears. Shocking fiction gives way to historical fact and reasonable future possibility. America habitually takes a lofty moral stance when making recommendations (or ultimatums) to other nations, but within our borders at all times one may find any number of persons or groups with motives for wiping out populations numbering from one to millions and those who would gladly accept the job. What has been lacking recently is a galvanizing force, a catalyst that reduces the gaps between the stepping stones of unthinkability, wishful thinking, feasibility, advisability, mandate, and reality. Like it or not, Americans are humans of the ordinary stamp, and humans, like it or not, are opportunistic omnivores, still subject to the worst effects of the law of tooth and claw. We are animals who possess a unique capacity for reason, a capacity so new that almost any of the older instinctual or learned behaviors interferes with its efficacy and primacy. Ancient hatred and fear were among the causes of death of that man in the gay bar parking lot. Reason, like a subordinate personality, was overpowered by the knee-jerk will to destroy.

The question of whether or not genocide is possible in America thus became moot for me. More to the point was the question, under what conditions could it occur? How much conniving among which individuals or groups would be required? How much could be kept from the public and for how long? To what degree would the public's acquiescence or complicity be required? How could manipulation of individuals, group dynamics, and mob psychology be used to create the required public climate? What role would the media play? These and many other questions rolled around in my head like marbles in a jar. All would have to be answered and couched in a believable, interesting story supported by a sound literary structure.

Tackling the Beast

For the sake of those who assume that some kind of cosmic order exists in the creation of a novel, I would like to say that *A Cry in the Desert* developed from a carefully wrought outline and was executed employing a host of preplanned writing techniques. I would *like* to say it, but it isn't true. I created no detailed written outline, and my application of writing techniques was as often instinctual as programmed. Rather, the book seemed to evolve through a thousand questions posed to myself and answers carved from the raw materials of fact and imagination, like pieces of a hand-carved jigsaw puzzle.

I had been writing in various forms since childhood. I had written novels employing both standard and experimental structure and had created works with many and some with relatively few characters. My settings had ranged from a single room to map bouncing. I had tried my hand at comedy and what passes for tragedy nowadays. And yet I felt myself unprepared. This project required that I employ writing techniques that had heretofore been for me simply names and examples from literature or college texts: time telescoping, sustained allegory, multiphased motivation, and so on. If I were to succeed, I would have to master the merging of reality and fantasy into a seamless whole. I would have to lead my readers from a believable and realistic "now" through gradually escalating horror to an unimaginable but equally believable "then." My characters would have to include a staggering range of social and ethical types, from street hustlers to bureaucrats, ministers, and psychopaths, each developed in his or her own right and recognizable in physical, ethical, and psychological traits while maintaining the essential qualities of individuality and reasonable reaction to internal as well as external stimuli.

I had thought myself quite cosmopolitan, well versed in the ways of humankind. After all, I had been raised in the country and had experienced the ways of "provincials." I had been to college, read mountains of print, lived in cities, taught youngsters and adults from varied backgrounds. I had been to Europe. I had not lived blindly, or so I assumed. I thought about writing, and the questions mounted, as did my apprehension and insecurity. What did I really know of medicine or the people who practice it? Of psychology? Of the tangled ways of business, religion, politics, the media, the military, or even of gay life and habits in more than a general way highlighted by limited but very specific experience? Sweeping generalizations, surface judgments, and stock characterizations would immediately mark me as an incompetent and lose for me any chance of getting my message across. I felt more humble than at any time in my life.

As I made notes and plans, I read, researched, talked to people as I had never done before. And I tried to listen, really listen, not to prepare arguments or encourage conversation, but to hear what was being said, what was not being said, the way in which it was said, why it was being said or avoided, the mannerisms of the person, his or her physical traits, tics, prejudices, foibles, and so on. I began to realize the incredible complexity involved in a single, apparently forthright statement, and I shuddered at the task I had set for myself. I couldn't manage it. Then, time after time, after admitting defeat, I applied that most consistently endearing and irritating of human characteristics: I worked around my inadequacies and forged ahead.

I am an avid notetaker. I fill notebooks to bulging with comments and observations, but when the writing actually starts, I find that I have either internalized their contents or I ignore them completely. I almost never refer to them, except to document hard facts. I write somewhat like a Navajo woman weaves. As a young Mormon missionary, I would watch in awe as one or another of those stoic women sat hour after hour creating in colored wool a design found no place except in her head. One thread at a time, color and spacing perfectly executed by nimble fingers until the completed rug stood before us on the loom. Some rug designs were simple; others were remarkably elaborate. (There are few crafts as complex and intricate as a Two Gray Hills rug with the design appearing in exactly opposite colors on the reverse side.) Admittedly, some rugs were sloppily made, their designs ill-formed, their colors gaudy with trading post yarn. Nevertheless, each rug came directly from the mind of the weaver, unalterable, inextricably woven.

Although it would pain my English and creative writing professors to hear it, my fiction writing technique is comparable to the way those women weave rugs. When it comes at all, the writing flows line after line, the content and continuity more intuitive than calculated. Line builds upon line, chapter upon chapter. Unlike one famous novelist who can create modular chapters in any order and plug them in where he desires, I begin at line 1, chapter 1 and finish with "The End." I edit as I go and rarely change anything afterward except for necessary technical editing. The whole picture remains in my head, as far as it exists, and it is fleshed out through the consistency of what has come before. This tends to drive editors crazy. "Just lop off a bit here and there," they might urge, "or expand this chapter a bit." Imagine my saying such things to a Navajo weaver: "Why don't you just move this figure up an inch or two." Her laughter would echo from Monument Valley to Tuba City. I don't mean to be difficult. It's just the way I function. *A Cry in the Desert* was tougher to write than most things I have attempted, due, in part, to this writing style.

Facts were few when I started writing. They grew more difficult to evaluate as time progressed. Theories and projections abounded and continually changed. I had to guess what would transpire. As it turned out, many of my guesses were accurate. Others were (and remain) plausible. As the story takes place between 1982 and 1984, it contains what were assumed to be facts at the time as well as speculations that the years would either confirm or refute. The book was never intended to be technical or used as a reference work. It is a novel, an entertainment with clearly didactic overtones.

For purposes of logistics, I telescoped events that might have taken a decade or more to evolve into a couple of years. Instead of approaching the crisis from a global aspect, I elected to show a microcosm, a few locations in the state of Nevada. I selected a handful of characters from the segments of local society that were most likely to be involved, directly or indirectly, in a plot to disfranchise, isolate, and annihilate a minority, exploring their motives as well as their actions. I attempted to present, wherever possible, a story without heroes, a story filled with gray areas and conflicting purposes. This, I believe, is the way life is. Even Botts, the monomaniac who is the pivotal agent of destruction, has variegated shades of determination, hesitancy, fear, and remorse. His complexity, along with the human inconsistency of other characters, makes the nightmare all the more real. Dr. Woodford, the nominal protagonist, considers himself impotent and a coward. All the characters have feet of clay. All, I hope, could be people one might know or see on the street anywhere in America.

There is a considerable amount of graphic violence and sex in the book. It was not my desire to exploit these for their own sake, but as a means of fulfilling my desire to provide the flavor of realism. Sex is what being homosexual is about. Otherwise, we are no different from anyone else. The potential effects of juxtaposing a segment of the population ostracized for its sexual orientation or practices with a medical crisis of this magnitude are the basis for the story. If the inclusion of these elements appears gratuitous or excessive within the context provided, I have failed in my intent.

Is Anybody Out There?

I finished the manuscript for *A Cry in the Desert* in late 1983 and confidently began looking for a publisher. Anticipating that the major houses would refuse to touch it, I concentrated on gay publishers. One after another rejected it. Some stated that the subject was outside their accustomed "target market," that is, mystery, sexploitation, or similar genres. Others felt that the treatment, though effective, was too strong, too militant, too graphic, too unsettling, and half a dozen other versions of "too." Oddly enough, every rejection letter urged me to try other publishers. Some provided likely candidates; in some cases, they recommended each other. All indicated that somebody was sure to publish my book. I began to doubt it. I felt alternately like Cassandra and a plain fool.

Since I was planning to move from Las Vegas to California and was going through a personal crisis or two, I decided to shelve the manuscript and concentrate on other projects. It lay in a box for two years. Then, when legislation was proposed in California for mandatory testing and quarantining of potential as well as confirmed AIDS victims, I thought it was time to try again. (Our detractors are both patient and persistent. They continue to try to disfranchise us, but so far they haven't succeeded.) By late 1986 the book had found a home, Edward/William Press, a small gay press in Texas. It (and I) came out in May 1987.

Fallout

All my fears and even a few of my hopes were realized in the reviews that followed. Naturally, they were all from gay publications. I was compared to the worst yellow journalists and to George Orwell. I was a sensationalist and an opportunist. Others called the book a masterpiece, a classic of gay fiction, and placed it among the "must reads." My writing style was praised and demeaned. I read the reviews with a curious sense of detachment. What mattered most was that the gay community was in the process of doing the unimaginable. In groups throughout the country, they were pulling together and embarking on programs of self-education and political activism that continue to amaze (and, in some quarters, alarm) the general population. I congratulate them (us) and hope that in some small way my writing has contributed to the will not only to survive but to prevail in the face of every adversity. As the potential for ultimate evil is always with us, we must never forget that we have the right and the power to be ourselves.

Terrors of Resurrection

"BY EVE KOSOFSKY SEDGWICK"

Michael Lynch chose to skip the MLA this year, having discovered that he is defatigable. But he wanted to be here today, if not in his own body then in mine, or at least in his own glasses, in mine. Since I consider Michael a genius—I heard bells when I met him, as I did when I first met Picasso and Professor James—I'm willing to collaborate with his puerile eagerness to publicize his book of poems, *These Waves of Dying Friends,* which will be published in January by Contact II Press, with monotypes by Douglas Kinsey, and will cost less than five dollars.

These Waves of Dying Friends records, occasionally even clarifies, meditations of a privileged, urban, gay, white American during the first years of the epidemic. It is largely elegiac, sometimes witty, sometimes bored with all these mortalities among friends. At the end, in a sequence set at the October 1987 civil disobedience on the steps of the Supreme Court, Lynch attempts to convert grief into anger, the passivities of mourning into directed political agendas. But if you ask me, there's a lot of elegy still in that call to arms. Today, I want to say a few words about the persistence of elegy, but not in Lynch's published collection. Instead, I want to go back to a poem he wrote fourteen or fifteen years ago, when disco bunnies like him localized their obsessions in giardiasis, not cytomegalovirus; in Donna Summer, not Susan Sontag; and in MDA, not AZT. It was, in their cultures, no less a complex time than the present. (Many people forget this.)

Lynch was localizing another obsession in the poem I want to read you and was even (for he *was* a junior colleague of Frye!) meditating an article on returns from the dead, or the apparent dead, in prose narratives. He thought himself fascinated by the dislocations that such returns spawn. But let his poem speak now. It counterpoints two voices, one composed of several short assertions, in parentheses (Lynch is fond of parentheses), and one including a single sentence, stretching out from the eighth line to the last, quite beyond comprehensible performability. The poem is called "The Terror of Resurrection."

The Terror of Resurrection

While you were away
I fought off cars
and the sweet orange capsules you left
for solace on the seat
(I knew cars are capsules
but the point was other
than what I knew).

Now that I've welcomed you back the terror
of resurrection
(catastrophe for the closest friends
must have been
that face
of what had been so grievingly safely bound
talking gently)

slaps against the hollow body

and the resurrection
(but theirs was nothing compared
to his:
facing the mourners' security
of well-done affection
and the disrupter himself jarred to find
himself this kind of disrupter)
of terror
(all around me old men,
goggled, swim)
must cover us now because in here
the air is shrinking
(I like this car, the pills.
I like having you back like this)
away.

Juvenilia like this, as we all know, relishes the easier props of death: orange capsules, sinking cars, suicide. Let's skip, then, the unparenthesized line and focus on two of the intrusions. The first imagines the reaction of friends when one whom they had bound and buried returns:

> (catastrophe for the closest friends
> must have been
> that face
> of what had been so grievingly safely bound
> talking gently)

The three Marys, the two men on the road to Emmaus, the friends of Lazarus, even Doubting Thomas doesn't face this catastrophe. Lynch probably did in his teens when his two favorite adults died. In grieving for them, he probably felt the guilt of welcoming their deaths: several years of ill health had wrecked his teacher aunt, and alcoholism had wrecked his father. "So grievingly safely bound"— "safely" cues what the analyst calls secondary gratification. And this safety, a pure component of true grieving, is what the returning person shatters.

The second insertion in the poem's counterpoint shifts to the consequent reactions of the returning person—let us call him a "him," first of all, and "the resurrectee." He too confronts catastrophe:

> (but theirs was nothing compared
> to his:
> facing the mourners' security
> of well-done affection
> and the disrupter himself jarred to find
> himself this kind of disrupter)

Again, the Gospel doesn't help us here. Despite his evocations, it doesn't seem to have helped Lynch either. For in the world outside its hagiographies, the resurrectee has every right to be jarred when his friends receive him not with rejoicing but with fretting. Let sleeping dogs lie; the dead remain in their shrouds.

At this point, I must invoke a gambit to distance us a little from Lynch's script. The problem with talking apocalypse or resurrection is their distance from lives as led. Let's talk in more proximate terms, terms more domesticated, certainly more secular. Let's talk of those persons in some of whose white cells a virus called HIV is replicating. We've learned how not to talk about the epidemic as a plague. Now let's try to talk about it, for a while, without the language of terror, of panic, of death, of resurrection, of apocalypse.

[Silence punctuated by efforts to speak that don't go anywhere.]

Well, we tried. There didn't seem to be much to say. AIDS is so firmly ligatured to death, in our framing of it, and to apocalypse, that we cannot easily locate alternatives. "A disease less apocalyptic," Paul Monette writes casually about some other one in *Borrowed Time.* Susan Sontag traces the American "need for an apocalyptic scenario" as a way of mastering "fear of what is felt to be uncontrollable." She observes the peculiar twist of the contemporary apocalypse, which always looms but never occurs. "It's not *Apocalypse Now,* but *Apocalypse from Now On.* "

The equations are so for-granted that we hardly need to hear them again: everyone infected with the AIDS virus is increasingly likely to eventually develop full-blown AIDS; opportunistic infections or a systemic wasting-away syndrome kills AIDS victims; terminal illness; mounting counts around the world; nearly always fatal, scientists say; no hope for a vaccine in the foreseeable future; no hope for a cure in the foreseeable future. People dying of AIDS. Dying of AIDS. Dying.

Now there have been some interesting developments in the past few years that challenge this ligaturing of AIDS with death and apocalypse. There is AZT. There are other antiviral or immune-boosting pharmaceuticals. There is aerosolized pentamidine, proving successful as a prophylaxis against pneumocystic pneumonia. There are diagnostic procedures that do not require the long wait for symptoms. There are strategies of early intervention. There is no cure and there is no vaccine, but increasingly AIDS seems potentially "manageable," analogous, say, to diabetes—at least for middle-class American adults who kick open the doors for access to these drugs, procedures, and strategies. How sensible some folks seem, then, when they shift the focus from death to chronic illness, from the apocalyptic AIDS to the proximate HIV disease, from AIDS victims to people living with AIDS, from palliative care to means for coping with reduced energies, from revising wills to demanding treatments.

To the degree that we shift the focus thus, we have shifted from the apocalyptic to the potentially manageable. This is very good news. There is, however, as Lynch and his activist cronies try to puzzle out, a very powerful resistance to hearing this good news. Lynch likes to say that the resistance is not confined to the Moral Majority or the editors of the *New York Times.* Resistance occurs in the doers of good, often genuine good, who overcome their distaste for marginalized sexuality or even marginalized drug use *as long as the marginalized are safely dying away.* Resistance occurs in medical workers, social workers, families of the diagnosed: how much we love you, how much we want to do for you, *since you are dying.* Resistance is most firmly entrenched in the media, where boilerplate lines such as "nearly always fatal" mar even stories about improved treatment prospects.

Resistance also occurs in people who accept their positive antibody test as a death sentence.

Lynch's poem may guide us here, at least to the degree that it invites us to contemplate the two catastrophes: (1) that of the well meaning who face a major disruption when their friend has returned from the apocalyptic equation's deathliness; and (2) that of the ill person who faces, may even be seen as causing, the disruptions that follow the abandonment of that equation. Violetta's is a safe, secure role; but what terror for an act 4 when she suddenly outlives act 3 and perhaps even dances away a few more years.

Is Lynch arguing that Alfredo, his dad, Annina, and maybe even Violetta herself are better off without such an act 4? No. Since he identifies shiftingly with all of them, he thinks they'd be happy indeed to delay the final curtain for another act. Or two. Or more. But since he identifies shiftingly with them all, he also thinks they'll have to face the unexpected terrors of this welcome rearrangement. He sees the challenge not as apocalypse now, nor as apocalypse from now on, but as getting the FDA and the NIH to expedite treatments, as working out manageable workloads with employers or thesis supervisors, as figuring out ways to cope with recurrent nausea, as figuring out ways to get down a *whole* peanut butter sandwich, as making time, not serving it.

Note

Before his death, Michael Lynch stipulated in a letter dated October 16, 1990, that his essay be titled "Terrors of Resurrection 'by Eve Kosofsky Sedgwick.'" He also wanted a note saying: "This piece was written by Michael Lynch to be delivered by Eve Kosofsky Sedgewick when he was unable to attend the conference for which it was planned": the Modern Language Association Meeting, New Orleans, December 1988.

It Can Happen: An Essay on the Denial of AIDS

The fiction writer and the journalist have different tasks. The fiction writer imagines a story and uses a voice to tell it. Journalists are supposed to report the facts. The chronicling of the AIDS epidemic has been for the most part left to journalists; the burden of truth, in the reportage, not in an imagined story. For a decade we have been forced to accept the horrific facts about AIDS glaring from the headlines, but we are not forced to read stories or see plays that confront us with the universal truths inherent in this life-and-death drama. Anyone writing fiction with AIDS as a theme will discover a reluctant, resistant, even rebellious audience. Why?

At the risk of bold generalization I'll answer this question with my own experience. When the AIDS epidemic began I was living in the San Francisco Bay area with my husband, who is an infectious disease specialist. We were immediately caught up in the maelstrom of this growing, mysterious tragedy. As a writer I believed AIDS stories were the ultimate in novelistic material. AIDS was a modern plague; it struck young people in the prime of their lives, was always fatal, and was sexually transmitted. The connection between sex and death was never so visible to the consciousness of a society, though most people wanted to shut their eyes to it. Naïvely, I decided to write a novel, hoping to open the eyes of many to this crisis and hoping to dispel the prevalent notion that AIDS is a gays-only disease. I wrote *Immune* in 1985 and 1986 while living in Zimbabwe, where AIDS afflicts men and women equally.

Immune is about a virologist living life in the fast lane in San Francisco in 1982. Suzanne Keller is a beautiful, successful, disillusioned workaholic who finds herself increasingly seeking escapist solutions to her despair. She is, like many of her generation, alienated and miserable in her private life and seeks therapy, where she finds seduction and drugs. She and her boyfriend, a Russian literature scholar, have an unhappy, open relationship, and although she is involved in the early research on AIDS, she doesn't question or change her own sexual relations. Led by her unscrupulous therapist, she plunges deeper into drug use and has affairs she can barely remember. Just when it seems a real love relationship might resolve many of her problems, she discovers that her now ex-boyfriend has the symptoms of AIDS. She commits suicide, opting for death as the ultimate escape.

The publication of this novel, for which both I and my publisher had grandiose fantasies of success, was met with disagreeable silence. Reviewers called it "disturbing," "depressing," "a scathing attack on modern society," and "of questionable taste." The critics, at least, were not interested in reading about the downfall of an attractive, successful professional, probably much like them. People who spread or had AIDS could not be viewed as *like them.* In the minds of mainstream Americans, AIDS must remain a disease of homosexuals and IV drug-users. The best example of this came a few months after my book was published. A screenplay writer telephoned me to say he thought the book had the makings of a good movie, but asked, "Do you think we could write a happy ending?" As recently as August 1991, a Hollywood agent told me what I had heard many times before: "No one in the movie business will touch this topic."

My novel was intended to unmask some of the illusions I think many people have about AIDS as a disease. The point was to show that no one is immune to the tragedy of disease or death. AIDS does not discriminate on the basis of sexual preference or moral inclination. As a disease AIDS is objective; the virus will live, multiply, and destroy cells wherever it finds a home. How one acquires the disease has unfortunately become like a trial at which the victim is eventually pronounced guilty or innocent.

In 1988 I was asked by an editor in Washington, D.C., to write a story about AIDS that involved "ordinary" people, by which he meant heterosexuals. He wanted a story with educative value to his upscale readership. I wrote the story that appears later in this volume, "The Federal Bureau of Blood Inspection." The issues of tattooing HIV carriers, creating special camps for them, keeping children with AIDS out of schools, turning people away from airports, and the like were hot items in the news. A few weeks later I got a polite note saying the story was rejected. I telephoned the editor, who apologetically said, "It's just too depressing. My co-editor can't accept the premise. He doesn't like it." The premise—straight, non-drug-using, young professionals have a baby who dies of AIDS—was too controversial. Once again I learned my lesson the hard way: stories about AIDS are not marketable. The idea that AIDS could happen to "us"—heterosexual, drug-free, middle-class America—is not an acceptable perspective on the disease no matter how sympathetic the characters are made to be.

Since lots of depressing, tragic stories are major successes in literature, why is AIDS the modern leprosy? Indeed, thousands of young men were dying of AIDS in the early 1980s, and it was not until Rock Hudson died that anything approaching national sympathy for victims of this disease existed.

The rejection of AIDS literature goes back to the first novel I know of with AIDS as a theme. *A Day in San Francisco* was written by Dorothy Bryant and published in 1982. It's about a mother searching for information at a Gay Pride celebration in San Francisco on what was then a new and mysterious disease. The mother finds almost nothing to warn the young men of potential danger, and she fears for her gay son. When I asked Dorothy about the response to her novel she said, "I got a lot of shit from the gay community. I got a lot of shit from the liberals, too." The response to her book was negative; she had said something gay people didn't like or didn't want to hear. She said blind conformity to the gay lifestyle was no less oppressive and restrictive than blind conformity to the constricted society she grew up with in the 1950s. No one wants to read AIDS stories about themselves; if people read an AIDS story and suddenly some identification with a character takes place they don't like it, they don't want to read anymore. This very aspect of a good story or an absorbing novel works against fiction with AIDS as a component.

One last example of an AIDS story that didn't get the readership it deserved. When I was writing *Immune* I was sent galley proofs of a book called *The Screaming Room* by Barbara Peabody, a true story of her taking care of her young son as he died of AIDS. Written in a fictional style, the book was engrossing, a page turner filled with the tedium of cleaning up vomit and diarrhea and the horror of watching her son grow old, demented, and blind. I was sure this book would be read by the millions of families who had suffered through this ordeal, but months later I heard it didn't sell. The readership wasn't there. AIDS stories are disturbing in ways that most people don't want to be disturbed. But people do want to be disturbed by novels of grotesque murders, terrorism, or cults that sacrifice children. Compared to the literary magnitude of the event (youths dying in their prime of an incurable disease) the literature of AIDS is scant. Why is it young men dying by the droves in wars has produced scores of novels, but dying of AIDS evokes silence?

A partial answer to such questions lies in how our society views disease, sex, and death. AIDS victims are separated into two groups: those who are "guilty" and those who are "innocent." The latter are the hemophiliacs and others who acquire the disease through blood transfusions, those given the disease by negligent health care workers, and children. The former are homosexuals and IV drug users. In other words, if you "ask for it" by having sinful sex or shooting up because you're addicted, then you deserve your fate. In our control-oriented, guilt-ridden society, AIDS is a failure of the individual. You are an "innocent victim" only if you get the disease due to circumstances beyond your control. Even so, "innocent victims" often report feeling guilty, as if they did something wrong, and they are certainly tainted with the stigma of AIDS after they're diagnosed. As Susan Sontag and others have pointed out, we view disease as something we've allowed to happen to us: we've failed to stay well.

Often the sick-well continuum is one of indulgence-deprivation: too much fat, sugar, caffeine, nicotine, alcohol, meat, and, today, stress. We are obsessed with the idea that what we do or don't do is the number one reason why we get sick or stay well. We are equally obsessed with the belief that if we get sick there must be something we can do about it. Failure to control desire is a serious character flaw, and failure to control a desire for pleasure, whether sexual or drug-induced, is worse. Overindulgence has become a disease (e.g., alcoholism); the medical model is being increasingly applied to psychology. Thus, almost everyone lives a guilt-ridden and hidden life of the flesh while striving to project the revived ideal of "Leave It to Beaver" and "Father Knows Best" lifestyles. There are no homosexuals or IV drug users in this picture. Look, for instance, at the few TV dramas that have attempted to depict the stories of AIDS sufferers. They have focused primarily on the families' acceptance or not of the protagonists' homosexuality. Concern is for the parents, particularly the moms. In one recent TV movie the AIDS sufferer never even appears as a character.

Our fetish with control over illness and health bolsters our resolve that death can be conquered, if not immediately, then someday. AIDS activists fall into this trap, often blaming the very doctors who are trying to help them: If we can't control our death, okay, but certainly the doctors can. If they don't have the solution, perhaps they're holding back information, perhaps they want their patients to die? The idea that doctors can't stop death is unacceptable. In general, as a society we idolize youth, we try to deny death, and we deify doctors. We see ourselves as powerful actors on the stage of a natural world subdued. Out of the "dark continent" AIDS appears, linking sex and death in a macabre, morbid drama, accelerating the aging of decades in a few short years. The disease ravages body and mind, and not just the minds of the victims, but the minds of anyone who confronts it. Our gods of science, in spite of the incredible speed with which the medical profession has advanced its knowledge of this disease, have failed us. They cannot cure AIDS. Yet. What we cannot control we deny. What we cannot deny we rationalize and justify. After ten years of government neglect in education and prevention, President Bush has the gall to tell Americans we should have compassion for AIDS victims. In our so-called enlightened society this hypocrisy is sickening.

For those who have been close to this disease, whether as a victim, a relative, a friend, a doctor, or a caretaker, the nastiest implication is that the disease is deserved. People who engage in "perverse" sexual acts or the "crime" of shooting up drugs deserve to suffer and die. AIDS is a punishment for sex or addiction. The underlying assumption of this view is that "AIDS will never happen to me." It is only the Ryan Whites, the "innocent" victims who don't fit into the crime-and-punishment scheme.

Why do some people believe AIDS could never happen to them? The answer: Because they never have sex. Whatever they're doing doesn't fall into the category of actual sex. Here an absurd pretense is clung to in the service of preserving the ideal image of clean, God-fearing, right-minded, upstanding Americans. It is no joke that entire books meant to educate readers about AIDS preach abstinence as the best way to avoid the disease. It handily solves the problems of birth control, abortion, and population control at the same time. This is the sort of fiction one doesn't find in fiction. Stories don't work if they're entirely unbelievable and impossible to imagine.

An April 2, 1990, article in *The Nation* by Bruce Fleming, recently returned from Rwanda, points out the provincialism of our North American view of AIDS. AIDS, disease, sex, and death are viewed much differently in Rwanda, where the problem of AIDS is much more serious. The same is true in Zimbabwe and many other African countries. Sex and death are not considered unnatural events. Disease and death are not alien or viewed as subject to human control. They are events that happen, part of the natural course of life. This is not to say that Africans like to get sick and die; they don't, but they don't view sickness and death as a failure to control events. Life goes on until it stops, without regard to individual volition. With respect to AIDS, the view of Rwandans, fatalistic though it may be, is also more realistic. The idea of abstaining from sex is utterly foreign to Africans, precisely because it is not realistic.

Silence in response to AIDS on the part of African governments (which really do not have the resources to fight the disease) comes less from denial than from the racist implications of the "African origin" theory of the HIV virus. The best scientific evidence indicates that the disease probably did originate on the African continent, but just as the outbreak of AIDS in the West began among homosexuals, a marginal and vulnerable group, the belief that Africa, a marginal and vulnerable continent, *gave* us this plague has implications Africans quite rightly reject. In addition, several African countries have embarked on much more comprehensive programs of education about the spread of AIDS than has the United States, with its vast resources. Still, in the words of a heroic young Ugandan musician, Philly Lutaaya, who died of AIDS in December 1989, "no one wants to be associated with AIDS." Philly Lutaaya spent the last months of his life traveling throughout Uganda in an effort to bring AIDS out of the closet and combat the shame of AIDS in his country. In an interview on "The AIDS Quarterly," he said he was not ashamed that he acquired AIDS sexually. His words to a crowd assembled for his last concert were, "It's okay to have AIDS. AIDS is not the end of the world."

In Zimbabwe I was constantly frustrated by the government's lackadaisical attitude toward AIDS and was forced to come face to face with my own Western prejudices that something could be done. I wrote a long, statistically detailed article on the AIDS crisis that was published in a major popular magazine. Many Zimbabweans read the article and agreed with the conclusions, but nothing was *done.* Giving people information does not necessarily change their behavior, not in Africa or here. I recently read a confessional article by a science writer who described how, even though she had multiple sexual partners and her partners had multiple sexual partners, she didn't always ask a man to use a condom when she had sex with him. She felt scared and guilty because she knew the risks, but she didn't always take precautions. According to the article, only 16 percent of sexually active women do. We may throw up our hands and say "people are crazy," but when we do we must include ourselves. In my novel and my stories about AIDS I've tried to do just this, and I'm irrationally optimistic that many readers will agree with me. In matters of powerful instincts and desires we don't have a lot of control.

What I have said about American society is not meant to be insulting; my intent is not to hurl criticisms but to share insights, many of which I've discovered by examining my own assumptions. I'm not advocating sexual promiscuity, drug-use, suicide or amorality. Rather, I'm advocating a critical analysis of our own barriers to understanding and compassion for the sick and dying, and a healthier respect for the objectivity, not the goodness or badness, of nature. I'm advocating the relinquishing of the idea that we, as individuals, can control the forces of nature. Fiction, I believe, has a powerful role to play in these pursuits. Stories are more powerful than good reporting, and this is why they are harder to read.

In Zimbabwe I heard many AIDS stories. One struck me as an especially tragic lesson. A man in his mid-thirties in a very high government position was diagnosed HIV-positive. He was a veteran of the Zimbabwean revolution, an athlete, and much admired. He was married and had children. The diagnosis was kept secret, but he eventually got sick and went to the hospital. He was in no immediate danger of dying and soon left the hospital. But his diagnosis was discovered and in a short time everyone heard he had AIDS. He was determined to show his friends and colleagues that he was still working and living. He decided to have a big picnic and invite all his friends. No one refused his invitation, but on the day of the party no one showed up. He drove to his home and shot himself through the head. AIDS did not kill him; the fear, silence, and betrayal of his friends did.

Early AIDS Fiction

It is easy to invent reasons why it took so long for AIDS to be thoroughly treated in fiction, the easiest explanation being there was no audience—and therefore no market—for AIDS fiction. Or, as this writer was told on numerous occasions, it was too soon to tell the story of AIDS—as though the epidemic would somehow run a neat course and have a nice conclusion. Or, as agents and editors mumbled, the critics and mainstream press would fail to review such work, thereby condemning it to obscurity and commercial failure.

The situation was not, however, so clear-cut. No, the reason many fiction writers were reluctant to approach the subject (if, indeed, they were) had little to do with such commercial considerations but had everything to do with artistic and, more significantly, psychological considerations. For most gay writers, AIDS was a profoundly *personal* reality—friends were dying of this mysterious malady with an alarming swiftness, and one knew almost nothing but this fact: withering illness and death. Was it an environmental toxin? Poppers? An infectious agent?

Nowadays, with the relative boom in knowledge about HIV disease and AIDS, it is difficult to recall the dark mystery that surrounded "the gay plague" in the early 1980s. But how on earth could anyone write about something so vague, so indefinite, so unknown, and, most important, so terrifying?

Writers *did* write about AIDS, however, and here we depart from the notion that AIDS fiction was somehow slow to appear. The idea that it took a long time for AIDS to be explored in fiction has its roots more in the parallel reality of AIDS denial/AIDS horror ("I can't believe what's happening is happening") than in actual fact, for as early as 1983 the mysterious plague was a burning theme in Dorothy Bryant's *Day in San Francisco* and Armistead Maupin's *Baby Cakes.*

Curiously, *A Day in San Francisco* might be considered the first AIDS-themed novel—though the disease had yet to be given its unfortunate acronym—the story of a mother dismayed by the illness and unrestraint rampant in the life of her son and his friends in San Francisco's gay neighborhood, the Castro. While condemned by the gay press for this novel, Bryant was, and is, a much-respected, widely read, accomplished novelist. The publication of her novel can hardly be thought obscure, and thus AIDS in fiction can hardly be considered absent during the early years of the epidemic.

In 1983 the *San Francisco Chronicle* published Maupin's immensely popular "Tales of the City" series, published in book form in 1984, in which one of the central characters loses his lover to AIDS. Once again, AIDS was a major theme in a widely read novel, hardly the stuff of obscurity.

My own novel *Facing It* was published in 1984 to surprisingly widespread acclaim in both the gay press and the mainstream reviewing media. Sales were astonishingly brisk for this first novel by an unknown writer. Generally credited as the "first AIDS novel" (because the book's theme is the epidemic), *Facing It* was the natural next step in the treatment of AIDS in fiction.

Also in 1984, Dan Curzon's novel *The World Can Break Your Heart,* in which the main character is touched by AIDS, appeared to some fanfare of its own. Concurrently, the theater, always able to respond "on the pulse," was the first place where AIDS art made its appearance, with Larry Kramer's play *The Normal Heart* and William Hoffman's *As Is.*

These early treatments—with their relatively strong critical and commercial success—certainly contradict any notion that AIDS was slow to appear in art or in fiction, or that it was somehow ignored. That it *seems* as if AIDS was ignored, unexplored, is the real curiosity, an almost amnesiac effect, as if, while reading about AIDS and writing about AIDS, everyone *felt* that nothing was being done. Was this perhaps an outgrowth of the helpless feelings aroused by AIDS, that it has remained so mysterious and unsolvable for so long?

This strange paradox—the real versus the ideal—has informed every aspect of the epidemic and continues to this day. AIDS science moves at a criminally slow pace but still faster than it ever has; while hundreds of thousands die worldwide just as clinicians call HIV a manageable chronic condition; while public service announcements declare that AIDS affects everyone, yet clearly it does not; while government spending reaches an all-time high and is nowhere near enough; while activists revolutionize treatment research that produces no results; while AIDS books that "do not sell" are published by the dozens.

To be sure, the literary heavy guns—gay and straight—were relatively silent the first half dozen years, until all at once there appeared Robert Ferro's *Second Son,* Christopher Davis's *Valley of the Shadow,* Alice Hoffman's *At Risk,* and Edmund White's (with Adam Mars-Jones) *The Darker Proof.* The reason for this, I suspect, is obvious. Much of writing and publishing is, for better or worse, dominated by New York. New Yorkers, and gay New Yorkers in particular, found themselves amidst the swirling maelstrom of death and dying, without even a moment to pause and reflect: Oh, this is an epidemic, how startling!

It was the dubious fortune of the west coast and the rest of the nation to have the time to look up and see the train racing down the tracks before it hit. Novelist Andrew Holleran, writing in *Ground Zero,* suggests that AIDS novels "weren't needed. . . . The truth was quite enough; there was no need to make it up" (13). Indeed, this was the obvious case in New York, where the epidemic struck like lightning. And it undoubtedly accounts for the fact that AIDS fiction appeared first from San Francisco, not New York, for it was in San Francisco that there was time enough to ponder the mysterious ailment that was yet a novelty out West while it consumed friends and acquaintances like a firestorm back East.

Surrounded by this sudden, wild hurricane of illness, many of our prominent gay writers—the Violet Quill and others—were naturally shell-shocked, unable to attain the observant, cool distance necessary for the creation of fiction. Perhaps, in sum, the problem is that no single, major masterpiece of fiction has yet emerged from the AIDS epidemic to take its place alongside the great novels of illness—Camus's *Plague,* Mann's *Magic Mountain,* Defoe's *Journal of the Plague Year*—giving rise, then, to a feeling that AIDS has not "really" been handled yet.

One supposes that, as Holleran also wrote in *Ground Zero,* "the act of writing seemed of no help whatsoever, for a simple reason: writing could not produce a cure" (16). But such a statement suggests that writing is ineffectual if it cannot be put to some immediate, practical use, and surely that is not true.

Fiction and drama hold the power to touch people at a level unreachable by news reports, statistics, prayers, or memorial services. To alert people to the calamity of AIDS by telling a story, to explore multiple facets of the epidemic and its wider meanings, to educate the general readership and influence public opinion through vivid imagery—these are all valuable and very real products of AIDS literature. AIDS writing may not produce a cure, but it can produce a climate in which a cure is more likely.

That was the early challenge of AIDS for fiction writers, and, unfortunately, it remains the challenge for fiction writers today.

Red Noses, the Black Death, and AIDS: Cycles of Despair and Disease

In his fascinating book on "mystical anarchists" and announcers of the Last Judgment, *The Pursuit of the Millennium,* Norman Cohn describes the extent of the bubonic plague, the Black Death, that devastated Europe—the first time—in 1348–49: "In the crowded towns the plague flourished ... overwhelming all efforts to check it; corpses lay unburied in the churchyards. It seems certain that ... this plague was incomparably the greatest catastrophe that has befallen western Europe in the last thousand years—far greater than the two World Wars of the present century together" (131).

Such devastation seems to dwarf our own "age of anxiety," rife as it is with "the experience of overwhelming insecurity, disorientation and anxiety" (Cohn 136). And such an experience often drives people toward "a collective flight into the world of demonological phantasies" (87). During the plague, some even believed that some demonic group "must have introduced into the water-supply a poison concocted of spiders, frogs and lizards—all of them symbols of earth, dirt and the Devil" (Cohn 87).

Cohn goes on to suggest that "the plague was interpreted, in normal medieval fashion, as a divine chastisement for the transgressions of a sinful world" (131). The plague brought out the worst and the best, everything from self-sacrifice to self-aggrandizement, from the Flagellants, who went around whipping themselves in public and were at one time supported by Pope Clement VI, to the cyclical revival of virulent anti-Semitism, blaming the Jews once more for everything. As Cohn again suggests, and as we shall see in our own "dark ages," "the civilization of the later Middle Ages was always prone to demonize 'outgroups'" (87).

But the broad religious questions remain. Is misfortune on such a grand scale deserved? How guilty should men and women feel in transforming a virulent disease into some form of divine scourge or punishment? Is there a cosmic equity at loose in the universe to account for the necessity in life of pain, suffering, and death? And if the Black Death revealed the wrath of God, what really was its cause—lack of faith, spiritual decay? Was the plague a sequel to Noah's flood? And if all interpretations tremble before such a fact of death, what then? Are we left bereft, victims of sheer chance, bitten by stray fleas and doomed?

In Peter Barnes's play *Red Noses,* which takes up the plague years and the search for scapegoats within them, Father Flote, a monk, decides to entertain the masses during the mayhem by donning a red nose and clowning around, as if acknowledging that such a procedure is as successful as anything else would be, and more productive than the Flagellants, the Black Ravens selling bodily fluids scooped out from the corpses, and the gold merchants clutching their coins. He attracts several disciples, and the Church goes along with it, hoping the Floties, as they're called, will take the people's minds off the Black Death that surrounds them.

Flote's mistake is to take his role too seriously. Once the plague shows signs of abating, he shows signs of leaping from being a mere clown to being a social revolutionary, a mystical leader opposed to the oppressive clank and clutter of the medieval Church. As the plague ends, the Church restores its command and authority, sees Flote as a thorn in its side, and has him and his disciples summarily executed. Barnes's upshot seems to suggest that institutions will do anything to survive. They will co-opt all outside movements, use them when necessary, distance themselves from them when necessary, and dismiss them if they threaten, in this case, the hierarchy of the powers that be. And history recycles itself: brave individuals come to the fore during grave crises, but then they must be eliminated during more placid times, so that institutions can reassert their authority and power.

It is perhaps a bit facile to draw connections between the Black Death and AIDS, but the connections still stare out at us as if they demand obeisance. In both instances, the public demands its scapegoats. As Ken Plummer explains, "AIDS has become a massive scapegoating device, neatly dividing the world into the 'guilty' and the 'innocent' by selectively blaming some of its 'victims.'. . . There is, however, nothing new about this scapegoating of those who are the 'victims' of disease; the Black Death scapegoated the Jews and massacred them"

(33). Exactly what kind of socially constructed, "cosmic" scheme can encompass AIDS? A divine punishment for the sexual revolution of the sixties? A strange eruption of chance once again in a world we like to think we're finally coming to grips with? Is this misfortune deserved? And are we once again driven to contemplate the fragile notions of a cosmic equity, a divine design hidden somewhere at the center of things? Interpretations can kill, and we'd better watch out who is making them. We can laugh at the merry bands chastising fate with their songs and red noses, but there are popes eager to reassert their all-too-earthly powers, and while we laugh, they may be brewing their own fatal potions of righteous wrath.

AIDS has become "the most talked about disease in recent history," Plummer maintains. "It has also come to assume all the features of a traditional morality play: images of cancer and death, of blood and semen, of sex and drugs, of morality and retribution. A whole gallery of folk devils have been introduced—the sex crazed gay, the dirty drug abuser, the filthy whore, the blood drinking voodoo-driven black—side by side with a gallery of 'innocents'—the haemophiliacs [sic], the blood transfusion 'victim,' the new born child, even the 'heterosexual'" (45). Such an iconography plays right into the public fantasies of Cohn's millennial history. And Plummer, quoting the psychohistorian Robert Jay Lifton, suggests that modern life seems to be "based on a 'new wave of millennial imagery—of killing, dying and destroying on a scale so great as to end the human narrative'" (34).

Out of such millennial iconography comes the backlash. "AIDS has come to serve as a most potent symbol for reaffirming the older orders that have been placed under threat in the mid-twentieth century," Plummer asserts (46). AIDS calls forth the apparent need to rally around the heterosexual family unit, whether that remains an actual description of present-day society or not. "As Foucault (1979) and others have argued," Simon Watney makes clear, "we need however to recognize that the image of the threatened and vulnerable family is a central motif in a society like ours for which the family is not simply a given object, but is rather an instrument of social policy" (59). Clinging to a perhaps outmoded social formation, we are bound to see enemies everywhere, and if we can't see them clearly, then we will invent our own folk devils to hold on to our defensive social position.

The art of demonizing outgroups is not, alas, a strictly medieval practice. Sander L. Gilman, in his classic studies of the stereotypes of sexuality, race, madness, and disease—*Difference and Pathology* and *Disease and Representation*—makes it quite clear that we all create stereotypes and that we all like to envision ourselves as healthy and "them" as diseased, so as to separate "them" from "us." In defining "their" difference, we thus define our "normalcy." As part of our own internal doubts and uncertainties, we project onto the world our fears and anxieties. The Other becomes the culprit "out there," so that we may preserve our sense of self and healthy balance "in here." "The human disposition to structure perception in terms of binary difference," Gilman argues, runs very deep, and once our self defines the Other as different, because of disease or sexuality or race, we have effectively erected the illusion of a boundary between "them" and "us" and rescued ourselves from "their" contamination (*Difference* 24). "Every social group has a set vocabulary of images for this externalized Other," Gilman suggests. "These images are the product of history and of a culture that perpetuates them. None is random; none is isolated from the historical context" (*Difference* 20). And once these stereotyped images grip the popular imagination, such "stereotyped stigmatized thinking can lead us to perceive whole sections of the population as somehow sub-human. And once that happens, anything can be done to them" (Plummer 47).

The process reveals itself in many of the portraits of AIDS patients that have appeared. These images embody the iconography of the syphilitic, of the melancholy and depressed soul. These patients are seen or photographed as isolated, distanced creatures, often black male homosexuals, already marginal figures in our society because of their race, their sexuality, their connection in the popular mind with criminal cityscapes and drugs. The films, articles, and interviews of such critics as Isaac Julien, Kobena Mercer, Richard Fung, Sunil Gupta, Marlon Riggs, Pratibha, and others make it clear that the public imagination seems to identify AIDS with gay people of color. Yet recent evidence shows that many people with AIDS are neither homosexual nor black—Plummer claims that "in North America [only] 25 per cent of all persons with AIDS are black" (30). Still, as Keith Alcorn has concluded, "AIDS has been portrayed as an *illness of difference.* This continual articulation of difference and non-difference is a crucial part of the rhetoric of normalization that dominates media coverage of AIDS" (74).

Art creates icons, and these icons fit our chosen images even as they distance them from us. Djuna Barnes sees the image as "a stop the mind makes between uncertainties" (qtd. in Robinson 164). Gilman explains that art, "whatever form it is given, is an icon of our control of the flux of reality" (*Disease* 2). Every icon embodies a communal act of interpretation, and all one has to do is look at the pictures of

AIDS patients to see how isolated we've made them, in what a frozen, emptied vacuum we've placed them, much like the demonizing tendencies of our distant medieval cousins.

Based on his findings about the spread of AIDS in Africa, where needles are used for inoculations again and again because they are expensive, Gilman builds an interesting (if still open-ended) case for the Western practice of inoculation as a significant contributor to the spread of the disease. This puts a different slant on the issue and reveals again the limitations of the iconography of the black, male, homosexual AIDS patient. It also reveals the underlying stereotyping of AIDS as a specifically African or Haitian disease, based on the notions of the supposedly prodigious sexuality of blacks.

What puts a certain apocalyptic spin on both Gilman's notions of the bipolarities of human perception and the sardonic, almost embittered look at polarities that rage between individuals and institutions in Barnes's *Red Noses* is Hillel Schwartz's view of the prominence of such polarities and threatening doubles in the final decade of a century, in this case the century before the second millennium. As Schwartz suggests in his tantalizing *Century's End: A Cultural History of the Fin de Siècle from the 990s through the 1990s*, "At centuries' ends people are prone to live by the doctrine of the excluded middle. . . . While we talk of transcending these polarities . . . we commonly oppose right-brain to left-brain talents, our artistic 'side' to our prosaic 'side. . . . to meet up with one's Double is to meet up with one's fate" (275, 210).

"Nothing is more punitive than to give a disease a meaning— invariably a moralistic one," Susan Sontag has written (62). As in medieval times, the AIDS disease can play to this manner of polarizing events, of stereotyping as part of human perception to begin with, and of distancing ourselves as "us" and "them" on a grander scale. And in America this "disease" is even more virulent, since we have for centuries polarized our view of the world, whether between Puritan and Indian, capitalist and communist, enlightened good and blackened evil, the legions of light and the hosts of darkness. Such a Manichaean worldview has been with us from the beginning—since the first cities on the hill—as part of what William Pfaff has called our "barbarian sentiments." Such a view continues to feed our conceptual construction of the world around us, and into its path all too easily has tumbled the onset of AIDS.

To the Manichaean mind the world remains a prison, created in a demonic chaos by someone other than God, some demiurge or evil Jehovah sprung from the hosts of darkness. Humankind is trapped in that prison, victimized by flesh and desire. We often seem possessed by some dark fate not of our own making. As Daniel Hoffman suggests, "Puritanism was perhaps as close to the Manichean as any Christian sect has come; the Power of Evil was acknowledged with the same fervor as the Power of Light. Indeed, it was a faith more pessimistic than that of the ancient dualists, for it made no provision for the goodness of man" (153). And in a wilderness where the devil's initiates lurked behind every tree, the Puritans could fashion their near-paranoia any way they chose.

Of course, recent scholarship in poststructural theory and semiotics has revealed the very real biases built into the nature of polarization. As Sacvan Bercovitch makes abundantly clear in *The Office of the Scarlet Letter,* personal interpretations invariably generate an either/or perspective and polarize problems or the meaning of events "into symbolic oppositions" (23). These polarities mutually sustain one another. In fact the tendency inherent in such a functional relationship is to privilege one of the polarities over the other: the Self, for instance, is far more "valuable" than the Other. Thus, by excluding a middle ground, such as the Puritans were accustomed to doing, the "in" group can easily castigate the "out" group and exclude them from the "proper" focus of their cultural and social constructions. What Bercovitch calls "a metaphysics of choosing" (88) solves the problem of either/or, in one fashion, by demonizing the outsider, thereby excluding him or her, and privileging the insider.

In the instance of ethnic identity in North America, the notion that it may be essentially fluid and subject to constantly changing, socially and culturally constructed categories clashes with the other cultural conception of race that holds "that race is biological, fixed by the genetic make-up of the individual and obviously marked by skin color" (Weiss 2). Missing from this conception is the more prominent vision that "marginalized groups can engage in a struggle with hegemonic forces and re-construct identity in their own terms, by redefining the standardized oppressive and singular (or totalizing) discourse about race" (Weiss 2). It is the first concept to which the popular imagination about AIDS and its "victims" seems to cling. It is the latter construction, beyond the status quo–seeking polarization of events and peoples, that needs to be emphasized.

Many American writers, beginning perhaps with Poe and Hawthorne, have looked out upon a dark, imprisoning world, occupied by isolated souls, diseased, victimized, and shunned. It would be easy to make a long list of such novels, including, for example, Norman Mailer's *American Dream* (1965), William Styron's *Sophie's Choice* (1979),

Thomas Pynchon's *Gravity's Rainbow* (1973), Joyce Carol Oates's *Bellefleur* (1981), Toni Morrison's *Beloved* (1987), Paul Theroux's *Mosquito Coast* (1982), Joan Didion's *Democracy* (1984), John Cheever's *Bullet Park* (1969), and John Updike's *Witches of Eastwick* (1984)—the list could go on and on. The tradition is a long one in our literature and shows no sign of ending soon.

The fiction of the last twenty years or so has only exacerbated this tradition, complete with ironic and dark fables, disrupted narratives, and tortuously self-reflexive tales, rife with paranoia, from the likes of Jerzy Kosinski, Don DeLillo, John Hawkes, and John Barth, to mention only a few. The age of such paranoid irony has produced its fair share of black comedies, its farcical satires and satirical farces, its picaresque parodies and grotesque conspiracies. And these forms, built squarely on our Manichaean literary visions and themes, have certainly contributed to the creation of such plays as Peter Barnes's *Red Noses*. Such visions, however, often build upon outmoded or stereotypical social and cultural constructions of race, marginality, sex, and disease. It would take more space than I have here to examine and explore the relationship between these dark fables and their darker counterparts.

A radical doubt in much of American literature disrupts all moral design. And the existence of AIDS certainly plays to this cultural script. "The sheer range and variety of AIDS commentary should alert us to the danger of any attempt to explain it in terms of any single, primary and all-determining causes," Simon Watney warns us, and we must continue to be on the lookout in literature and the media for certain "ideological concerns, which transform AIDS into a *malade imaginaire*—the viral personification of unorthodox deregulative desire, dressed up in the ghoulish likeness of degeneracy" (61, 60). The counterattack is already upon us from the likes of Jesse Helms and others who brand as obscene that potent brew of the AIDS legacy and art in Robert Mapplethorpe's provocative photography.

AIDS has already invaded the theater and fiction. It may suffer the same fate as much of our Manichaean literature, being viewed as one more confirmation of the evils of this world, coupled with the American dread of sexuality entwined with self-reliance and individualism. Barnes seems correct when he suggests that, in these days of plague, institutions preserve themselves first before rallying to the needs of individuals. In any case, we should be aware of the warnings epitomized in *Red Noses* and always on the alert to identify the seemingly psychological necessity of our own self-preservation through our stereotyping of the Other. These are deep-seated, dangerous responses that are all too human—and will continue to supply the heart of our images of ourselves and in our fiction in the 1990s and beyond.

Works Cited

Aggleton, Peter, and Hilary Homans, eds. *Social Aspects of AIDS.* Philadelphia: Falmer Press, 1988.

Alcorn, Keith. "Illness, Metaphor and AIDS." In Aggleton and Homans, 65–82.

Bercovitch, Sacvan. *The Office of The Scarlet Letter.* 1970. Baltimore: Johns Hopkins University Press, 1991.

Cohn, Norman. *The Pursuit of the Millennium.* New York: Oxford University Press, 1970.

Gilman, Sander L. *Difference and Pathology: Stereotypes of Sexuality, Race, and Madness.* Ithaca: Cornell University Press, 1985.

———. *Disease and Representation: Images of Illness from Madness to AIDS.* Ithaca: Cornell University Press, 1988.

Hoffman, Daniel. *Form and Fable in American Fiction.* New York: W. W. Norton, 1961.

Pfaff, William. *Barbarian Sentiments: How the American Century Ends.* New York: Hill and Wang, 1989.

Plummer, Ken. "Organizing AIDS." In Aggleton and Homans, 20–51.

Robinson, Douglas. *American Apocalypses: The Image of the End of the World in American Literature.* Baltimore: Johns Hopkins University Press, 1985.

Schwartz, Hillel. *Century's End: A Cultural History of the Fin de Siècle from the 990s through the 1990s.* New York: Doubleday, 1989.

Sontag, Susan. *Illness as Metaphor.* Harmondsworth: Penguin, 1983.

Watney, Simon. "AIDS, 'Moral Panic,' Theory and Homophobia." In Aggleton and Homans, 52–64.

Weiss, Wendy. Unpublished report on a cultural diversity workshop with Elliott Butler-Evans, Wheaton College, May 1991.

■ JAMES W. JONES

The Sick Homosexual: AIDS and Gays on the American Stage and Screen

The view of homosexuality as an illness has a long history, reaching back at least to the Middle Ages. Since the Enlightenment, physicians have concerned themselves more and more with this "aberrant phenomenon," as they most often saw it, and the modes of same-sex love as disease were increasingly codified in both medical texts and legal writ throughout the nineteenth century.[1] Our own century has seemed to take larger strides away from a perception of same-sex preference as a sickness, beginning with Magnus Hirschfeld's theory of a "Third Sex," developing with Kinsey's statistical report, and progressing to the abolition of homosexuality per se as an illness by the American Psychiatric Association in 1973. The homosexual of the early twentieth century has become the gay person of the present.[2] However, the link of same-sex love and disease, be it physical or psychological, although weakened over the course of the 1960s and 1970s, never evaporated. AIDS has revivified it in the popular, heterosexual mind and within gay culture. (I am using "gay" in its popular meaning of referring to homosexual men and homosexual male culture.)

The conceptual relationship between homosexuality and illness however, has clearly changed: AIDS has moved the focus from the psychological to the physical. No longer is homosexuality an expression of psychological degeneracy; now its physical expression can lead to death.[3] AIDS has given new impetus to the link between homosexuality and disease but has not reforged that bond between the two which the gay liberation movement of the twentieth century has broken. There exists, however, a dangerous cultural dialectic within which this disease operates: on the one hand, the media and works of literature seek to spread the truth as to the nonidentification of homosexuality and AIDS; and on the other hand, the myths about homosexuality and illness reinforce that link. This dialectic operates within the plays, films, and television dramas produced for the American stage and screen since 1984.[4]

The works under discussion here are the following:

PLAYS

As Is, William Hoffman, 1985. Rich has AIDS and, with the help of his ex-lover, Saul, confronts the disease and copes with his family and friends. Unlike the next two works, this play does not end with the protagonist's death. Instead, Saul climbs into Rich's hospital bed for some safe sex.

The Normal Heart, Larry Kramer, 1985. A fictional retelling of the development of the Gay Men's Health Crisis in New York City. The plot centers on Ned's fight against both a heterosexist bureaucracy and a homosexual minority that ignores the dangers of AIDS.

Safe Sex, Harvey Fierstein, 1988. A trilogy of one-act plays dealing with the effect AIDS has upon different men in the gay community.

FILMS

Buddies, Arthur Bressan, 1985. A gay man is assigned as a "buddy" to a gay man who has AIDS. Over the course of the latter's dying, they build a friendship that improves the quality of both of their lives.

Parting Glances, Bill Sherwood, 1985. Nick, the best friend of Michael, one of the main characters, has AIDS, but the disease plays a minor role. The relationship between these two predates Nick's illness and only intensifies the feelings of love Michael has for him. Yet Nick realizes Michael has also made a commitment to his lover, Robert, and the film's slice-of-life tone weaves all three characters and their relationships together while resolving none of them.

Longtime Companion, Norman René, 1990. The film follows a group of gay men and a heterosexual female friend from the first mention of "a mysterious disease affecting homosexuals" in the *New York Times* in 1981 through 1989. Along the way, the audience watches several of the men die and others deal with being diagnosed HIV-positive. The men and the woman form a community of support and love as they move from fear to sorrow to activism.

TELEVISION DRAMAS OR EPISODES

An Early Frost, 1985. Michael discovers he has AIDS, returns to his family, and reveals both his illness and his homosexuality to them. Each of his relatives eventually comes to accept him. In the end, he returns with his lover to their apartment.

An episode of "Brothers," 1985. One of Joe's former football teammates reveals that he is gay and is dying of AIDS. Both Joe, who is heterosexual, and his gay brother Paul provide support for their friend. This character is the only African-American man with AIDS in any of the works discussed here.

An episode of "St. Elsewhere," 1984. A married politician learns that AIDS is the cause of his night sweats and fatigue. He reveals his affairs with men to his physician, but he chooses to keep everything a secret from his wife, children, and constituency.

An episode of "Designing Women," 1987. A gay friend of the four main characters reveals he has AIDS and asks the women to decorate a room at a funeral home that serves many gays who have AIDS.

Episodes of "St. Elsewhere," 1987–88. Portions of several episodes involve two lovers: Kevin, who is HIV-positive, and Brett, who has AIDS. The episodes portray Brett as a patient, Brett and Kevin as young men in love, and, finally, Brett's death, all of which are subjected to the homophobia of those around them, an emotion only slightly tempered by the love offered by a few heterosexual acquaintances and family members.

An episode of "L.A. Law," 1987. A gay man who has AIDS is convicted of second-degree murder in the mercy killing of his lover, who had begged him to kill him so as to end the misery he was suffering while dying from AIDS.

An episode of "The Trials of Rosie O'Neill," 1990. A gay man who is HIV-positive is brought to trial for murdering his lover who has AIDS. Whereas the gay man in the "L.A. Law" episode fights the system, this man wants to be found guilty so that he can receive the death penalty and more quickly end his life. Rosie, his public defender, delivers an impassioned summation in which she attempts to make the jury see him as someone like them. She has realized this herself because she has had to deal with the trauma of being tested and awaiting the test result. The defendant, however, is convicted of manslaughter when his HIV status is revealed to the court.

An episode of "Law and Order," 1990. Currey, a gay man who is HIV-positive, is prosecuted for helping gay men with AIDS commit suicide. The district attorney secretly provides the defense with information that leads to Currey's acquittal, because he believes "Currey's already under a sentence of death. That's as much payment as anyone could ask for."

Our Sons, 1991. A very conservative mother from Arkansas renews contact with her gay son because he is dying from AIDS. In the process of their reconciliation, the man's lover and his own mother, who had initiated the reunion, also confront their own estranged relationship.[5]

In *Illness as Metaphor,* Susan Sontag writes: "the most truthful way of regarding illness—and the healthiest way of being ill—is one most purified of, most resistant to, metaphoric thinking" (3). While each of these works seeks to disseminate a truth about AIDS and about the gay person with this disease, they also, because they employ the filter of fiction, deal in metaphor. On the textual level—what the characters do and say—these works do not reestablish an identification between homosexuality and disease. Homosexuality is not presented as the cause of AIDS. Indeed, such argumentation along these lines is brought forth in *An Early Frost* and *The Normal Heart* and is explicitly refuted. Although each work centers on a male homosexual who develops AIDS, this character is not a person suffering the fruit of his aberrant desire but rather a person with AIDS (PWA) who happens to be gay. This line separating the PWA from the diseased gay proves thinly drawn. While traceable within the plot line, it sometimes is erased within the broader contours of the work's sketch of a gay person with AIDS.

In creating a fictional presentation of a gay man who has AIDS, these works draw also upon the myth through which AIDS and homosexuality are (mis)understood. It is within this realm of myth that the link between homosexuality and illness is made, and the bridge between them is AIDS. The myth of homosexuality itself as an illness steps out of the closet into which the gay liberation movement of the 1960s and 1970s and even the psychiatric-psychological establishment had sought to place it (Bayer 15–41). Their attempts were unsuccessful, since the link between homosexuality and disease continued to exist in the public mind, to at least some degree. By killing gays, AIDS has breathed new life into the beliefs many have held despite any medical or psychological assertions to the contrary.[6] These beliefs are voiced within several of the works, by heterosexual and homosexual characters. The question arises in *An Early Frost, Our Sons, The Normal Heart,* and *As Is* whether this disease represents the deserved retribution of nature (God/life) upon an existence led contrary to the rules of that higher power. In addition, the fear of infection from contact with the PWA reminds one of the myth of the contagion of homosexuality.[7] Thus, the nature of the disease, as a viral agent that, at least in the United States and western Europe, has affected mainly male homosexuals, plays upon two aspects of the mythology about homosexuality. But these dramatic works, to a greater

(*The Normal Heart, An Early Frost*) or lesser degree (*Parting Glances, As Is*), attempt to break the power of myth with the force of truth.[8]

In doing so, these works (with the exception of *Parting Glances,* in which Nick is just one part of the slice of gay life presented on screen) take on a didactic intent, aiming to enlighten their audiences as to the truth about AIDS. Clearly, enlightenment is needed. At this point, the works demonstrate degrees of difference, both in their presentations of the gay PWA, and, more important, in their perceptions of the gay PWA. These degrees of difference originate in an important distinction that exists between the works produced on stage or on film and those for television.

Each television drama, whether it be the TV movies *An Early Frost* and *Our Sons* or the episodes of TV series that are devoted to gay characters who have AIDS, portrays that character within a largely heterosexual social group, usually composed of family and health care professionals. Michael of *An Early Frost* leaves his lover to return to his parents' home. There his mother and, eventually, his physician care for him. In the process, other members of his family also come to grips with his situation as a gay PWA. In *Our Sons,* the gay man dying of AIDS begins reconciliation with his long-estranged mother, thanks to the efforts of his lover and his lover's mother.

The bisexual politician confronts and chooses to hide his disease within the hospital setting of "St. Elsewhere." In the final minutes of the episode, we hear a media report that he has indeed revealed his illness, but his sexual orientation remains unspecified. In "L.A. Law," "The Trials of Rosie O'Neill," and "Law and Order," the gay man with AIDS has been forcibly removed from his gay environment after he kills his lover. On "Brothers," a former teammate explains his impending death to Joe, one of the two heterosexual brothers in the series. By placing the character within this largely heterosexual situation, the TV dramas create a discourse in which the character becomes the victim. The victim testifies as to the tragedy set upon him by forces beyond his control. He pleads for understanding and for acceptance. In fact, the gay person has practically no other role available within the TV world, for until the 1987–88 season no network series, since AIDS has become a social issue in the West, has integrated a gay or lesbian character into its cast, thus relegating the gay person to the status of outsider. Such a character can only appear as a guest in the lives of the series' main characters, of interest for the problem he or she represents and the solution the main characters can supply or at least help this outsider find.

This mode of presentation is essential to the didactic intent which these dramas pursue. These programs aim at enlightening the viewing public about this disease and the fact that those afflicted with it are not inhabitants of some netherworld but rather the relatives and friends of the audience. The problem of AIDS in television is represented as a lack of understanding, of both insufficient enlightenment and empathy. The heterosexual social group within which the gay person finds himself, because it is the majority, represents the world to which he seeks access. He desires the love of his family, the care of doctors and nurses, the comfort of friends. They all possess what he needs, and in order to acquire them the homosexual must become the victim. He must go before them and present his case, bringing to bear the facts, hoping that the truth which he supplies will unleash their good will.

TV clearly exists to transmit information, disguised as entertainment or as news, to the majority of society, a majority that is heterosexual. AIDS and homosexuality in these TV dramas function within a discourse constructed by the heterosexual majority to explain to that majority what exists beyond its boundaries. Simon Watney describes the limitations and dangers of that discourse:

> We should, however, recognize that there is no *intrinsic* connection between HIV and gay men or their sexual behaviour. In this respect the continued homosexualization of HIV disease in the face of all the worldwide evidence concerning the diversity of social groups already affected strongly implies that the notion of HIV as a "gay plague" in fact protects heterosexuals from facing up to something which they find even more frightening than AIDS—namely, the diversity of sexual desire. . . . The logic of this resistance *requires* that AIDS should continue to be taken for granted as a "gay plague." This is not an accidental description, but protects and strengthens a fantasy of supposedly "natural" heterosexuality, attacked on all sides by sinister perverts. (33, 35–36)

This discourse, aimed at a majority, nongay audience, can frame that explanation only within the parameters of a "problem play." In the problem play, a character personifies the problem (e.g., rape, child abuse, alcoholism), and the solution lies in bringing out the facts surrounding the problem. The audience, according to this TV discourse, will attain an enlightened consciousness through these newly acquired facts and apply them to reevaluate and indeed reshape reality.

This is not an inherently futile exercise, despite the fear of homosexuality that, as Watney describes, may at least in part fuel these depictions. These television dramas about AIDS (for that is what they are really about) stand within a long tradition of the discourse about homosexuality in the twentieth century. From the turn of the century until the late 1960s, a major genre in the literary depictions of homosexual characters was precisely the problem play (or novel) in which the homosexual confronted a heterosexual society hostile to his or her sexual orientation and was forced to explain the reasons for that orientation and to defend the right to love someone of the same gender. Here, too, the works aimed at enlightenment, trusting in the power of "truth" to bring about acceptance of the homosexual minority by the heterosexual majority.[9] Tolerance and understanding were the goals of the problem play and remain so today. The medium of TV, aiming as it does at the widest possible audience, can only pursue such goals.

Such goals are not modest. They are, however, limiting. These TV dramas evoke sympathy for the plight of the gay man afflicted with a deadly disease, but their reach extends no further. In so doing, they perpetuate what problem plays throughout this century have done: they reinforce the category of homosexual (here the homosexual with AIDS) as Other. His presentation as a victim portrays him as a supplicant for sympathy. Sympathy can only be granted by someone who stands outside the victim's predicament. By operating within the genre of the problem play, these dramas set up categories that separate the very spheres they hope to unite, namely the gay PWA and the heterosexual majority. In them, the homosexual becomes the victim and thus remains the unknown, a being apart from "us," the same, the comfortable known—in other words, *those not in danger.* These dramas desire sympathy, which, however, can turn into pity, and both emotions can be granted as well as rescinded. The gay PWA pleads, hoping for a sympathetic ear. But the position of supplicant reinforces the status quo that has maintained a separation between the heterosexual and the homosexual. This is the dilemma of the discourse within which these dramas operate: that the sympathetic listener, when placed in danger—perhaps from fear of infection by the PWA—will turn away.

Two episodes of network television series take steps away from being purely problem plays, but still function within the television discourse. An episode of "Designing Women" demonstrated the farther-reaching ramifications of AIDS by placing equal focus on the popular link between gay males and disease and on the question of providing condoms in schools. The gay PWA plays a small role; he mostly serves to instigate debates about AIDS as just retribution for "abnormal" lives and about the issue of providing condoms to adolescents. The episode ends with his funeral, where it becomes clear that the young man's request to the women has been fulfilled (namely the redecoration of a room at the funeral home that serves many gays who have died). The ending is tragic and affecting precisely because we are made to realize that we must deal not only with a disease that, as yet, cannot be cured, but also with a prejudice that too often refuses to be changed by factual information.

In its final year (1987–88), *St. Elsewhere* also tried to expand the television discourse on AIDS. An ongoing character, Brett, had AIDS, and portions of several episodes detailed his stays at the hospital, his short-lived period of renewed health, and his relationships with his lover, parents, and doctors. Over the course of the television year, the writers demonstrated a change in their own understanding of AIDS and of this gay PWA. Early on, Brett's lover, Kevin O'Casey, tells Brett's doctor that he has tested HIV-positive and says, "I can't have a physical relationship with anybody ever again." He intends the statement to force Brett's doctor to realize the human cost and pain of living with the disease, something this homophobic male doctor has refused to do. (Instead, the doctor avoids Brett as much as possible and treats him from a cold—and safe—distance.) Kevin's statement belies the truth for those who test positive, as the "safe(r) sex" campaigns have attempted to teach. Although in this episode both the gay PWA and the gay man who is HIV-positive are portrayed within the traditional context of sympathy, in a television world that believes a dose of "truth" can cure social ills, later episodes attempt to transcend those limitations.

After Brett has recovered from a bout of pneumonia, he and Kevin celebrate by taking a walk during the afternoon. They are holding hands, an act that in itself is something new for the TV screen and enrages a passing carload of teenage boys. These boys attack the men, shouting antigay epithets, including references to gays as spreaders of AIDS. Again, the issue of homophobia is dramatized, for Brett's and Kevin's mere existence and their identification as gay men provoke a vicious response from a homophobic society. The episode depicts the increasing acts of violence directed against gay men due to the fear of AIDS among the heterosexual majority.

"St. Elsewhere" also focused attention on heterosexuals with AIDS and on the question of medical ethics in the treatment of AIDS patients. Two doctors in the series, both male, were affected by AIDS (through HIV infection): one received a blood transfusion that transmitted the virus to him, and he left to work with AIDS patients in California; the other was Brett's physician in the episode just discussed. This doctor could not deal with his own homophobia and traded his patient to a female doctor for one of her troublesome patients. Before that, however, he accidentally pricked himself with a needle he had just withdrawn from Brett's arm, and he later tested positive for the virus. Instead of intensifying his homophobia, this accident caused him to empathize more deeply and genuinely with Brett's situation. It also ushered him through a "born-again" religious experience, after which he became a more caring person and a proselytizer for his Christian cause.

The final episode in which Brett appears shows him extremely ill and almost totally alone. His relationship with Kevin seems to have ended, the disease being the reason for the breakup. His parents do not accept his homosexuality. A nurse proves most understanding and compassionate. She provides friendship and comfort for him. The doctor who infected himself with the virus from Brett's blood appears in the final scenes of Brett's life. He tells him that Brett can gain inner peace by renouncing his homosexuality. Although weak, Brett responds: "That would be going against what I am. Leave me alone." Later, the doctor returns and finds Brett lying on the floor, too sick to crawl back to bed. He repeats his offer to help Brett make amends with God. Brett tells him: "Kevin gave me the strength to embrace my own nature. You don't know how hard it is to live in this society and to be gay. To have to deal with your parents, your friends, the people at work. I've had to struggle so hard to live the way that I want to live and I've accepted that. And now I'm dying. Tortured by AIDS. And you say that even God will reject me if I don't reject myself. I'm never going to find any peace."

That speech is an indication both of the progress the television discourse on AIDS has made and of its limits. Those lines boldly describe the life of gays and of PWAs today, and by describing, they challenge the viewers' sense of justice, of fairness, and of compassion for their fellow men and women. At the same time, they evoke the traditional plea for understanding and sympathy. The most recent television movie to deal with this theme, *Our Sons,* continues such a presentation. Again, the gay man is presented to a presumably heterosexual audience within the parameters of heterosexuality: a young, white, upwardly mobile man (who is also gay and has AIDS) and his relationship—or lack of it—with his mother remain the focus. His status as victim continues unabated despite the somewhat heightened level of anger at uncaring social institutions expressed by the gay lovers. While *Our Sons* reassures us with its message of familial reconciliation, that reassurance is hardly long-lasting. After all, the gay son is near death; the issue of homosexuality, which his mother still seems to see as the real disease (and AIDS simply as its most recent manifestation) can be glossed over until it conveniently disappears. That is rather typical of the television representation of gay men in general: they exist singly as well-dressed creatures who inhabit tastefully decorated spaces but never share an on-screen kiss with another man.[10]

The aforementioned episodes of "St. Elsewhere" portray aspects of gay life and of the lives of gay PWAs with more honesty than other network television episodes have (witness its attempts to deal with gay-bashing, homophobia in the medical profession, the attitudes of right-wing Christians, and its portrayal of a gay relationship); yet, because the focus remains on a gay man with this disease (clearly to be expected in a hospital drama), the presentation of the gay PWA ultimately appeals, as always, to the sympathetic American sense of fair play. The episodes make a strong appeal, but sympathy, as pointed out earlier, is a dangerous emotion, for it does not necessarily lead to concrete acts of help or of social change to improve the conditions that evoke sympathy.

This change in the television discourse on AIDS was noted by Laurie Stone, media critic for the *Village Voice:*

> Now, on news shows, the people principally at risk are seldom presented from the inside. Rather, they're mostly portrayed as the problem with which the rest of the population has to contend. The focus of empathy has switched to health care workers and other "innocent" victims of AIDS: babies and the transfused. On daytime TV, the focus is just as skewed. Last month, CBS rebroadcast *An Enemy Among Us,* a Schoolbreak Special about a high school boy who gets AIDS from a blood transfusion. And on the two soaps running AIDS stories, *Another World* and *All My Children,* both sufferers are young, white, sexually conservative women. . . . The women AIDS sufferers are depicted as complete victims. They're good, clean, white girls. Once they get sick, they don't even consider having sex.

Stone concludes with the pointed observation:

> By omitting the majority of sufferers, daytime TV suggests that people who got AIDS because of their lifestyles—getting high and getting laid—aren't as deserving of empathy. One large effect of these shows is to give the majority audience—which is heterosexual, non–IV drug using, and aware, at least, of safe sex—a vehicle for venting anxieties about illness. In the absence of stories depicting high-risk groups, this venting trivializes real pain. It's like dramatizing the Holocaust without mentioning Jews and spotlighting only the group Hitler might have gone for *next.* (58)

The remarkable interest that three television series have shown in the topic of assisted suicide for gay men with AIDS is a logical but insidious progression in the depiction of gay men with AIDS on American television. The choice of this particular theme encodes a dangerous message to gays, be they HIV-positive or -negative. The mere use of this topic, I maintain, keeps alive the dangerous links between homosexuality and disease as a deadly threat. Just as in the early years of AIDS in America, when gays first "killed" other gays by infecting them with HIV and then spread that infection so as to threaten the non-gay population (so goes this myth), so are gays now "killing" gays with AIDS by means of assisted suicide. What is to keep that murderous trend from turning into yet another lethal threat posed by gays to the non-gay majority?

At the end of the "Law and Order" episode discussed earlier, Currey, the man who helped others die, is acquitted. He tells the district attorney: "This was not a prosecution, but a warning." Indeed it was: not a warning about the legal and moral ramifications of mercy killing, but a warning from the nongay majority to gay men everywhere to cease and desist the threat they pose. The threat is not just from AIDS. The links of homosexuality to disease and the assumption of AIDS as a literal manifestation of that inner disease make it clear that what really threatens the majority is homosexuality itself. It is no accident that a story about gay men with AIDS is framed as a story about mercy killing, for in so doing it allows the majority voices in the drama to express dismay, sympathy, and tolerance while at the same time serving the aims of homophobia —that is, eliminating gays. And, marvelously, it is another gay who is eliminating them. Not only have gays brought death to each other by transmitting HIV, but now they are even speeding up the dying process.

In contrast to these television episodes, the gay person with AIDS in stage dramas and independently produced films is integrated into a social group composed largely of other gay people. What Vito Russo writes about the lack of gay characters in Hollywood films is also true of the lack of Hollywood films that deal with the AIDS crisis: "We [gay people] have no acceptable context, and it's up to us to create one by being more open about who we are. Then we will be people and not targets" (73). This defines the difference between the ways in which Hollywood films (in which gay men with AIDS do not exist) and television programs represent gay men and gay men with AIDS, and the ways in which plays and independently produced films can deal with the subjects. In the latter, gay people are able to live truly gay lives, with all the multiplicity and veracity of interactions the term implies.[11]

The film *Buddies* centers on the relationship that develops between a buddy and a gay man dying from AIDS. *As Is* and *The Normal Heart* move almost exclusively within gay worlds in which the person with AIDS is nurtured, cared for, and loved by his family of choice, and only tangentially, if at all, by his family of blood. *Parting Glances* provides a bridge between those works that place the person with AIDS within a largely homosexual or largely heterosexual social unit. For most of the film *Buddies,* Nick remains in his apartment and willingly suffers the ministrations of his friend Michael. When he leaves to attend Robert's going-away party, where gays and non-gays will mix, he becomes the object of a heterosexual's curiosity about death. For this man, Nick exists only as a body being consumed by disease, and Nick lashes out at him, refusing to allow him any power over his life.

These plays and films share a common presentation of the gay person with AIDS. In each he is a *resister.* He refuses to succumb either to the conception of disease as due punishment or to the conception of the diseased as tragic victim. In these works, the character emphatically does not equal the disease. The break of identification between disease and diseased is made possible because the character exists within a social realm that provides support for him as an individual, separate from any status he might acquire as a patient. Here it becomes clear that the differing expectations or aims placed upon the various media make possible a different presentation of the gay character with AIDS. The plays and films under discussion here were not intended to appeal to the broadest possible public. Their didacticism centers not so much on education about the "truth" of a disease (which that of the TV programs does) as it does on the very manner in which a social unit, ranging in size from two lovers to the fictional equivalent of the Gay Men's Health Crisis, deals with an epidemic.

Because these works seek different goals from those of TV programs, they contain different structures. They place the character within a gay milieu where he can gather strength and courage. They deal with fears of contagion, of continued erotic desire, of death in a way that other works cannot. They build community among the outsiders of society. Whether they issue a call to arms, as *The Normal Heart* and *Buddies* do, or empower gay identity with continued life, as *Parting Glances, As Is,* and *Longtime Companion* do, their portrayals of the gay person with AIDS as resister, not victim, stem from that conception of gayness each work carries: its marriage to a community of friends and beloved, and its divorce from a facile identification of sexual orientation with disease.

In these works, the gay person with AIDS is not intended to evoke sympathy from the audience; instead, he functions as a sympathetic character. He represents the conduit by which audience identification is channeled, not into a catharsis of spirit that evaporates in the dark of the theater, but rather into the audience's active participation within the real world outside so as to effect social change. The audience should join in the resistance that the character on the stage or the screen offers. Although AIDS clearly dominates three of these works, none of them can be termed a problem play in the way that the TV dramas can. Whereas the TV dramas end in a catharsis that does not cleanse emotions but rather purges hope, these films and plays build hope and deny death a futility. They do so because they set the gay person with AIDS inside a gay milieu.[12] In these fictional works—as in reality—that gay milieu provides love, caring, and comfort. Such emotions serve as the basis for courage in the face of death and sustain a vision of gay identity in the face of hostility from those who fear the disease.

On stage, the image of the gay PWA as resister continues, although the portrait is receiving greater nuances and variations in recent plays. The number of stage works has increased dramatically since 1988—just as the number of television episodes or specials on gays with AIDS has significantly decreased (for, after explaining the "problem," there is little left for television to do but wait for its audience's sense of fair play to go into action). It would be impossible to discuss all the recent stage works that in some way deal with gays and AIDS; therefore, a work by a rather well-known writer will serve as an example.

Harvey Fierstein's recent trilogy of one-act plays, *Safe Sex* (which had a brief run on Broadway), does not deal with people with AIDS but with people affected by the fear of contracting AIDS and with people who have lost someone they love because of AIDS. The first play concerns a man frozen into immobility by his fear of contracting the virus. Manny closes this play, "Manny and Jake," with the words: "I can't change. I can't. So, I'll sit. And remember. And pray for everything else to change. And when it does (and it will) I'll remember how to kiss. [*He smiles.*] And I will give only what I choose to give. And I'll take only what I want from that which is offered. I will give and I will take without fear of small print or hidden clauses. [*Quiet ecstasy.*] And I will kiss . . . ! I will kiss having learned nothing" (24).

The second play, "Safe Sex," also centers on this fear but shows how love, and caution, can break that fear. Mead and Ghee, former lovers, argue, while teetering back and forth on a seesaw, about whether it is safe to have any kind of physical relationship again. Mead wants to renew their relationship, but Ghee is unable to conquer his fear of AIDS. In perhaps the most moving speech of the play, Ghee (who was played by Fierstein) recounts at length what life was like before AIDS, ending with the statement: "And we were invisible. Nobody knew who we were for sure. We were the great chic mysterious underground and I loved every minute!" (57). He continues with a depiction of the stark contrast of today's situation:

> And then came now.
> Different times. Now we enjoy politics and argue sex. Now they know who we are. . . . Now they see us everywhere: hospitals, classrooms, theaters, obituaries. . . . Now when they tell lies about us we answer back. We've found our voices. We know who we are. They know who we are. And they know that we care what they think.
> And all because of a disease. A virus. A virus that you don't get because you're Gay, just because you're human. We were Gay. Now we're human. . . .
> I love you more now than I did on our most carefree day. . . . And it's impossible. . . . We can never touch as before. We can never be as before. "Now" will always define us. . . . At last we have Safe Sex. (57–58)

At this point, Fierstein breaks out of the immobility that seems to have overtaken Ghee and trapped him as surely as it has trapped Manny. Ghee turns "accusingly to the audience" and says, "Safe for them!" And Mead responds by simply, yet emphatically, making two statements: "You're not [alone]" and "I love you" (58). After Ghee is convinced that externals may change but love can make all things possible, the two men balance the seesaw on which they have been having this discussion by walking toward the center. They meet in the middle, and the play ends with their embrace. Part of the reason that Ghee conquers his fear, while Manny does not, is that Ghee *is* part of a gay community—if only a community of two—while Manny is completely alone. His conversation is really a series of monologues and of talking past each other that occur between him and a man who would like to have a brief relationship with him.

The third play, "On Tidy Endings," deals with the lover and the ex-wife of a man who has recently died of AIDS. While they divide the household, they express their anger at and love for each other. Both win understanding, and love makes life possible and meaningful—as always in Fierstein's plays.[13]

Longtime Companion continues the tradition of presenting gay men with AIDS or HIV as resisters. Here, indeed, one might call them resistance fighters, for the film depicts their battles to save each other, to nurse lovers and friends, to cope with the effects that the health crisis brings into their lives. Within the film, it is by and large gay men who *must* do this, for the nongay majority does not have to, believing it is not "at risk."

As Dennis Altman points out in *AIDS in the Mind of America,* AIDS has revitalized the gay movement, providing it with new structures and new goals (82–109). These changes in the movement reflect changes taking place within the conception of homosexual identity. Richard Mohr skillfully delineates the essential role that sex has played within the definition of that identity. A homophobic society has made possible such a definition only within the realm of erotic exchange. Avenues of openness have been, for the most part, closed to gay people. Mohr argues that AIDS should be seen as the best argument yet for combating homophobia and for integrating gays into society, since the removal of the stigma is the only solution to a situation that perpetuates death by denying the right of gays to exist. Such a view is debated in *Buddies* and, to some extent, in *As Is.* (Television has not found a way to frame such a discussion and still suit its goal of serving the "majority" audience).

Larry Kramer's play *The Normal Heart* centers on the need to redefine gay identity. The debate between a definition according to sexual acts and a definition according to sexual orientation is argued by Mickey, one of the activists involved in the crisis center organized by gays, and Ned:

> MICKEY: I've spent fifteen years of my life fighting for our right to be free and make love whenever, wherever. . . . And you're telling me that all those years of what being gay stood for is wrong . . . and I'm a murderer. . . . Can't you see how important it is for us to love openly, without hiding and without guilt? (103)

Ned later tells Bruce, who has replaced Ned as the leader of the crisis center Ned founded:

> The only way we'll have real pride is when we demand recognition of a culture that isn't just sexual. It's all there—all through history we've been there; but we have to claim it. . . . And until we . . . organize ourselves . . . into a united visible community that fights back, we're doomed. That's how I want to be defined: as one of the men who fought the war. Being defined by our cocks is literally killing us. Must we all be reduced to becoming our own murderers? Why couldn't you and I . . . have

been leaders in creating a new definition of what it means to be gay? (114–15)

Kramer stands clearly on Ned's side in this argument, but that position does not deny the importance of sex to gay identity; it merely seeks to remove it from a position of dominance. Gays have responded to this life-threatening disease by affirming, not by sacrificing, a gay identity. Altman quotes from a letter written to a gay newspaper: "Yes, I believe AIDS means death. Death of an old lifestyle and *creation* of a new one. This is the full circle of love. The gay community is the healer of our times, because of your total freedom to be creative, your joy in living and the enormous opportunity to love yourself and others at this time. This is the healing of our times" (193). The revolution proves not to have been in vain. It was not about more and better orgasms, but about the ability to love.

This love is not limited only to those within the gay community. Heterosexual friends, especially women, supply comfort and compassion in *As Is, Parting Glances,* and *Longtime Companion.* Emma, the heterosexual doctor in *The Normal Heart,* bridges the gay and medical communities. The play ends with the embrace of the two brothers, Ned and Ben, one homosexual, the other heterosexual. Kramer's work makes the point that everyone, regardless of sexual identity, must cooperate in facing this crisis, for all of us belong to the same tribe. Yet Kramer's work, like the others, makes abundantly clear that one part of the tribe has been forced to shoulder the responsibility for the struggle and for the blame. Thus, although the formation of the gay community within these fictions (as in the real world) demonstrates many very positive and hopeful aspects, it also runs a great danger: that AIDS is seen as a gay disease, for those afflicted with it in these works are gay and their support comes from a largely gay community. This separation of the diseased gay from the healthy straight, no matter how fallacious, pushes all gays back into the category of Other, of stigmatized outsider.

In addition, since AIDS is a disease that at present in the U.S. largely affects gays, gays run the risk of being reassigned to the purview of the physician. Altman mentions the influence felt within the gay movement: "The most obvious impact of AIDS has been to produce a new professional leadership in the gay movement, one whose legitimacy is based on expertise rather than on either movement experience or popular representation. Increasingly, people with medical and scientific credentials come to speak for gays in public forums, and to influence the overall direction of the movement" (103). Michael Lynch, however, points up the more dangerous aspect of this remedicalization: "Like helpless mice we have peremptorily, almost inexplicably, relinquished the one power we so long fought for in constructing our modern gay community: the power to determine our own gay identity. And to whom have we relinquished it? The very authority we wrested it from in a struggle that occupied us for more than a hundred years: the medical profession" (qtd. in Altman 137). Richard Mohr draws the most frightening conclusion: "Worse than the further degradation of gays in America would be a general, and not easily reversed, shift in the nation's center of gravity toward the medical model and away from the position, acknowledged in America's constitutional tradition, that individuals have broad yet determinate claims against both general welfare and social ideals. The consequences of such a shift would be that people would come to be treated essentially as resources, sometimes expendable—a determination no less frightening when made by a combined father, colonel, and doctor than by a fearful mob" (62). With the assignment of gays to the status of diseased creatures, the return of the pink triangle may not be far away.[14]

Clearly, this is a danger that exists today, however latent. Intensified calls for mandatory testing signal the fear that AIDS evokes. The works discussed here conceptualize the sick homosexual in a variety of ways, but some of these concepts add to that danger. The TV dramas do so by presenting the gay PWA as a tragic figure. As such he evokes sympathy, but not empathy. He becomes the Other, the recipient of pity granted from a position beyond threat of contagion and beyond direct involvement—which could lead to true understanding. But when he becomes the murdering angel of supposed mercy (on "L.A. Law," "The Trials of Rosie O'Neill," and "Law and Order"), then, I maintain, fear overwhelms any message of empathy which the episode may seek to transmit.

The Normal Heart, As Is, Buddies, and *Longtime Companion* set the sick homosexual directly within the medical environment and argue for understanding the disease as a tragedy. The gay person retains his individual humanity as well as his membership in the gay community, a realm that remains beyond the television screen. Yet that very community, as I have argued, represents a danger of assigning the gay person with AIDS, and, by extension, all gays, to the category of Other. This danger does not arise in *Parting Glances,* although a strong sense of gay community exists within the film. The reasons for this can be found in the fact that AIDS is not medicalized, AIDS is not the "problem" of the film, and Nick does not die. Yet even in a film where AIDS speaks in so subdued a voice, what Dennis Altman writes about the disease remains true: "AIDS haunts us both asleep and awake, and it changes not just our behaviour but our very conception of who we are and our belief in ourselves" (24).

These films, plays, and television dramas contribute to that conception and to that belief. Like the disease itself, their presentations and the perceptions they evoke bring with them certain dangers. In contrast to the disease, however, the majority of these works—in particular the plays and films—affirm the human spirit.

Notes

1. Some important works from the increasing amount of writing on the history of sexuality and sexual orientation include the following: Boswell, *Christianity, Social Tolerance, and Homosexuality;* Faderman, *Surpassing the Love of Men;* Foucault, *The History of Sexuality,* vol. 1: *An Introduction;* Licata and Petersen, *Historical Perspectives on Homosexuality.*

2. Some works detailing this process or various stages of it include the following: D'Emilio and Freedman, *Intimate Matters;* Katz, *Gay American History* and *Gay/ Lesbian Almanac;* McIntosh, "The Homosexual Role"; "Sexuality in History," a special issue of *Radical History Review,* ed. Padgug.

3. Simon Watney, in *Policing Desires,* makes this plainly evident in his analysis of the public discourse on AIDS (and especially gays with AIDS) in Great Britain and, to some extent, the United States. Barry D. Adam also discusses this in an unpublished article "The State, Public Policy, and AIDS Discourse."

4. There have been short articles in such mass-circulation magazines as *Newsweek, People,* and *TV Guide,* and more in-depth pieces in *The Advocate, Christopher Street,* and *New York Native,* whose audience is largely made up of gay and lesbian people, but I have found little discussion in scholarly journals of the representation of gay people with AIDS in fictional works for the stage or screen. See, for example, Newton, "Sex, Death, and the Drama of AIDS." A special issue of *High Performance* devoted to AIDS as a cultural phenomenon analyzes several works on this theme. It is a different matter for representations in literature.

For a cursory analysis of the treatment of AIDS on recent nonfiction television programs, see Goldberg, "What Is TV Telling Your Patients?"; Kroker and Kroker, "Panic Sex in America."

5. This is, of course, an incomplete list, but it provides an overview of works that deal with gay men with AIDS or HIV and that have appeared on the American stage and screen.

The following works also treat this topic:

FILM

Men in Love (Marc Huestis, 1989).

TELEVISION DRAMAS OR EPISODES

"Biographies" of Rock Hudson and Liberace, 1989 and 1990. An episode of "Lifestories," 1990. Episodes of "thirtysomething," 1990–91. *Andre's Mother*, 1990. *People Like Us*, 1990.

DRAMA

Falsettoland, William Finn and James Lapine, 1989. Several plays have also been published recently, including Chesley, *Hard Plays, Stiff Parts;* and Patrick, "Pouf Positive." Osborn's collection *The Way We Live Now* includes the plays discussed here, along with several others. It provides an excellent overview of the ways in which this genre can deal with gays and AIDS.

6. Particularly helpful in understanding this linkage, which also involves the psychological processes of repression, resistance, and transference, is Watney's article "Psychoanalysis, Sexuality and AIDS."

7. This fear of contagion lay at the root of the reaction evoked by Rock Hudson's kissing of Linda Evans on "Dynasty" when later it was revealed that Hudson had AIDS. Viewers expressed shock and indignation (along with many other emotions) when they were informed that Evans was not told that Hudson was ill. The hysteria surrounding this incident, however, far exceeded any risk to Evans.

8. See these histories of lesbian and gay literature: Austen, *Playing the Game;* Foster, *Sex Variant Women in Literature;* Levin, *The Gay Novel;* Loeffler, *An Analysis of the Treatment of the Homosexual Character in Dramas Produced in the New York Theatre from 1950 to 1968;* Sarotte, *Like a Brother, Like a Lover.*

9. I leave aside the question of whether such a "truth" exists.

10. Witness the public outcry by conservatives and fundamentalists when "thirtysomething" dared to show two gay men in bed together. ABC–TV capitulated to the demands and refused to allow that episode to be rebroadcast in the summer reruns (1990).

11. For an analysis of Hollywood's reluctance to tackle this theme, see Natale, "And the Cameras Rolled On."

12. A major exception to the film portrayal of gays with AIDS is *City in Panic*, a "slasher" movie in which gay men with AIDS, along with others, are viciously murdered. The murderer, a woman with AIDS, leaves her signature on each—a huge M carved into the victim's body. Released only in video by Trans World Entertainment, the film has been attacked by the Alliance for Gay and Lesbian Artists in the Entertainment Industry as "totally irresponsible" (*The Advocate* 13 Oct. 1987: 17).

13. A new type of stage work dealing with gay PWAs has evolved from the need of those diagnosed with AIDS or with ARC or those who are HIV-positive to use the theater as a vehicle for coping with and changing their world. Well known from many performances in San Francisco and from a shorter version broadcast on PBS in 1987 is "The AIDS Show." Among other works are a similar effort by the New York City People with AIDS Theater Workshop, which performed in January 1988, and Michael Kearns's performance piece "An Actor Confronts AIDS." Although differing in style from more traditional plays such as

The Normal Heart and *As Is*, these works share with them the creation of a gay community and the presentation of the gay PWA as a resister.

14. A few examples of the many repressive steps that have been suggested and even acted upon out of fear of contagion: mandatory HIV testing of all foreigners who wish to reside in Bavaria (the home of the National Socialist party from the early 1920s through the end of World War II) and mandatory testing of all foreigners who wish to reside in the former Soviet Union. If the person tests HIV-positive, he or she is denied permission to reside in the country in question and is asked to leave. In the United States, the suggestion most reminiscent of Nazi tactics was given by William F. Buckley (and printed in the *New York Times*): "everyone detected with AIDS should be tattooed in the upper forearm, to protect common-needle users, and on the buttocks, to prevent the victimisation of other homosexuals" (qtd. in Watney 44).

Works Cited

Altman, Dennis. *AIDS in the Mind of America.* Garden City, N.Y.: Doubleday, 1986.

Austen, Roger. *Playing the Game: The Homosexual Novel in America.* Indianapolis: Bobbs-Merrill, 1977.

Bayer, Ronald. *Homosexuality and American Psychiatry: The Politics of Diagnosis.* New York: Basic Books, 1981.

Boswell, John. *Christianity, Social Tolerance, and Homosexuality.* Chicago: University of Chicago Press, 1980.

Chesley, Robert. *Hard Plays, Stiff Parts: The Homoerotic Plays of Robert Chesley.* San Francisco: Alamo Square Press, 1990.

D'Emilio, John, and Estelle B. Freedman. *Intimate Matters: A History of Sexuality in America.* New York: Harper and Row, 1988.

Faderman, Lillian. *Surpassing the Love of Men: Romantic Friendship and Love between Women from the Renaissance to the Present.* New York: William Morrow, 1981.

Fierstein, Harvey. *Safe Sex.* New York: Atheneum, 1987.

Foster, Jeanette. *Sex Variant Women in Literature.* 2d ed. Baltimore: Diana Press, 1975.

Foucault, Michel. *The History of Sexuality, Volume 1: An Introduction.* Trans. Robert Hurley. New York: Vintage Books, 1980.

Goldberg, Marshall. "What Is TV Telling Your Patients?" *AIDS Patient Care* December 1987: 46–47.

High Performance 4 Sept. 1986; special issue on AIDS.

Katz, Jonathan. *Gay American History: Lesbians and Gay Men in the U.S.A.* New York: Thomas Y. Crowell, 1976.

———. *Gay/Lesbian Almanac: A New Documentary.* New York: Harper and Row, 1983.

Kramer, Larry. *The Normal Heart.* New York: New American Library, 1985.

Kroker, Arthur and Marilouise. "Panic Sex in America." *Body Invaders: Panic Sex in America.* Ed. Arthur and Marilouise Kroker. New York: St. Martin's Press, 1987. 10–19.

Levin, James. *The Gay Novel.* New York: Irvington Press, 1983.

Licata, Salvatore J., and Robert P. Petersen, eds. *Historical Perspectives on Homo-sexuality.* New York: The Haworth Press, 1981. [Originally published as a special issue of the *Journal of Homosexuality* 6, nos. 1–2 (Fall/Winter 1980–81)]

Loeffler, Donald L. *An Analysis of the Treatment of the Homosexual Character in Dramas Produced in the New York Theatre from 1950 to 1968.* New York: Arno Press, 1975.

McIntosh, Mary. "The Homosexual Role." *Social Problems* 16 (1968): 182–91.

Mohr, Richard D. "AIDS, Gay Life, State Coercion." *Raritan* 6.1 (Summer 1986): 38–62.

Natale, Richard. "And the Cameras Rolled On: Why You Are Not Seeing Movies about AIDS." *Village Voice* 20 Feb. 1990: 67, 70.

Newton, G. "Sex, death and the drama of AIDS." *Antioch Review* 47.2 (Spring 1989): 209–22.

Osborn, M. Elizabeth, ed. *The Way We Live Now: American Plays and the AIDS Crisis.* New York: Theatre Communications Group, 1990.

Padgug, Robert A., ed. "Sexuality in History," a special issue of *Radical History Review* 20 (Spring/Summer 1979).

Patrick, Robert. *Untold Decades: Seven Comedies of Gay Romance.* New York: St. Martin's Press, 1988.

Russo, Vito. "Russo on Film." *The Advocate* 25 Sept. 1990: 73.

Sarotte, Georges-Michel. *Like a Brother, Like a Lover: Male Homosexuality in the American Novel and Theater from Herman Melville to James Baldwin.* Trans. Richard Miller. Garden City, N.Y.: Doubleday, 1978.

Sontag, Susan. *Illness as Metaphor.* New York: Farrar, Straus and Giroux, 1978.

Stone, Laurie. "Illin': AIDS and the Soaps." *Village Voice* 8 Mar. 1988: 58.

Watney, Simon. "Psychoanalysis, Sexuality and AIDS." *Coming on Strong: Gay Politics and Culture.* Ed. Simon Shepherd and Mick Wallis. London: Unwin Hyman, 1989: 22–38.

———. *Policing Desires: Pornography, AIDS, and the Media.* Minneapolis: University of Minnesota Press, 1987.

Facing the Edge:
AIDS as a Source of Spiritual Wisdom

"Something is happening on Earth," declare world religious leaders expecting the millennium. So declare eco-activists concerned about nuclear waste and ocean pollution. So declare evening news anchors reporting events in Eastern Europe. So declare AIDS activists demanding better education and better treatment.

What that "something" is varies from group to group. Some people see doomsday upon us. Some see a utopia about to rise from the toxic ashes of the last two thousand years of Western history. The coming of the Age of Aquarius, global awareness, realignment of morphogenetic fields, a quantum leap in evolution, Teilhard de Chardin's "collective consciousness," paradigm shift—all are mythometaphoric expressions for a significant change in the way human beings relate to themselves and to Earth.

What all probably have in common is the consciousness that, at least in the Western calendar, we're approaching a critical year as both the century and the millennium turn over. This moment, however, is not merely an artifact of time-keeping. As the Age of Aquarius hype in the late 1960s anticipated, the year 2000 will mark a change in the Sun's position in relation to the star patterns tracked by astrologers, a change that has been anticipated for thousands of years. And the critical moment is not only in the macrocosm. Life on Earth is undergoing ever-increasing change and stress. Indeed, it has become a commonplace that with new weapons technologies the world is on the brink, that the population is filling up the planet, that the advent of new social, scientific, and cultural paradigms is happening faster than any of us can keep up with, and that modern-day disasters threaten to reverberate throughout the world.

One of those disasters that seems to be generating ever-new repercussions is the spread of the HIV virus and AIDS. Within gay culture—where, in America, AIDS has struck the hardest—new philosophies, theologies, psychologies, and moralities are developing in response. The onrush of thought about AIDS appears in fiction and nonfiction alike, from books to tabloids and from scholarly journals to skin magazines. Some of the responses are dark and pessimistic (Tim Barrus, for instance, called his book *Genocide: The Anthology*); some are positive and hopeful (Norman Shealy and Caroline Myss called their book *AIDS: A Passageway to Transformation*). Some are funny (David Feinberg's *Eighty-sixed*); some are disturbing and outrageously sexual (Dennis Cooper's *Closer*); and some are deeply moving (Paul Monette's *Borrowed Time*). All these are part of the rapidly expanding genre of gay and lesbian literature.

What was once a hidden, anonymously written collection of sometimes lyrical and literary works (like E. M. Forster's *Maurice*)—though more often seedy, embarrassingly written and embarrassing stories of unhappy sex published by secretive small presses—has blossomed into a full-blown literary genre published proudly by both successful entrepreneurial "desktop publishers" and mainstream houses. Big New York publishers now have whole gay and lesbian imprints in both front and back lists. There is a network of gay, lesbian, and feminist bookstores across the country with trade journals targeted to them and book review journals targeted to their customers.

The "something" happening in gay literature is not only the rise of the genre but, more important, the development of the gay or lesbian hero—the individual who faces ordeals, struggles against all odds, usually armed only with truth and virtue, and ultimately conquers, often through a hard-won belief in himself or herself and a willingness to be honest. Gay heroes run the gamut from Billy Sive in Patricia Nell Warren's ever-popular *Front Runner* to John Preston's pop-adventure superheroes to 'Bel, the enlightened E.T., in my own *Secret Matter* to Robert Ferro's and Paul Monette's literary psychological protagonists. The appearance of the gay hero—in detective, mystery, science, and romance fiction as well as in literary novels and, especially now, in novels about AIDS—indicates a major change in the way gay and lesbian people experience themselves and their roles in life.

Homosexuals have been taught that they should be failures, pariahs, unloved and unlovable outcasts. Instead, in experiencing gay culture, at least some of them have discovered that they and their friends are wonderful, loving, generous, and certainly interesting and entertaining persons, loved by many people around them. They've discovered they can be courageous in the face of danger and hardship, self-sacrificing in tragedy and disaster. In a word, they can be heroes. And an early step in their hero's journey is the accomplishment of the ordeal of "coming out."

The appearance of these characters in fiction redefines how the gay public in turn defines itself. By reading of such heroes' journeys, other gay people develop courage and conviction and faith in themselves and in the truth of their own experience so that they can come out—that is, so that they can break the self-perpetuating prophecy of the homosexual as miserable pervert and create a new archetype. Thus has gay life been transformed by the change in consciousness experienced by male and female homosexuals in America in the 1970s and 1980s.

As Toby Marotta has documented in *The Politics of Homosexuality,* the gay counterculture arose out of the larger counterculture (84–91, 308)—of which so much was said in the early 1970s by hopeful and insightful thinkers like Theodore Roszak and Charles Reich (one straight, the other gay). That counterculture was committed to "revolution through consciousness change." The 1970s idealists truly believed they could remake the world by changing the way people thought about themselves. For a variety of reasons the counterculture dissipated as it became incorporated into mainstream American society. Countercultural ideas and values, especially cynicism about government and patriotism and concern about health and ecology, were carried into mainstream thought. For that very reason, it has been difficult to trace the results of the consciousness revolution.

Yet in one small segment of the counterculture—the baby boom homosexuals—there is clear evidence of the success of revolution through consciousness change. With the advent of feminism and the rise of a popular and political gay liberation movement, homosexuals began to think differently about themselves in the 1960s, and their world changed dramatically. For gay people, at least in principle, that revolution meant being honest and eschewing phoniness. And it changed the country's image of homosexuality and lesbianism and gave rise to a new political and economic minority, in fact redefining the very notion of minority status.

The rise of lesbian and gay liberation is the evidence for revolution through consciousness change. And this dynamic works in the individual's life just as it does in society's. This dynamic is reinforced, propagated, and refined in the fiction and nonfiction of the gay literary genre.

One might object that the appearance of AIDS in the 1980s refutes the claim for the success of gay liberation, that AIDS proved the error of homosexual freedom. But we must look to the very structure of the mythic hero's journey that is the core theme of the literature as well as the pattern of the social movement. Coming out and assembling together in a gay subculture was only the first step of this journey. What Joseph Campbell calls the "crossing of the first threshold" *necessarily* led to the "road of trials," along which obstacles would have to be overcome to find enlightenment and herohood with which to return bearing boons. In myth, suffering is one of the trials along the journey, less often a punishment than a visitation of God. (Christians interpret the passion of Jesus, for instance, as evidence of his saintliness, not of his sinfulness. The Roman persecution of the early Church is seen as "baptism by fire" that proved and strengthened the faith.)

AIDS, then, can be understood not as a punishment from God but as a challenge and an instruction. To cite but one example: the health crisis has brought a new interest in relationships. While not entirely adopting the so-called heterosexual model of fidelity and monogamy, criticized as institutionalized ownership of women, gay men have sought to improve the quality of their emotional lives. Thus, one of the fastest growing subgenres of gay and lesbian literature is the relationship book: for example, Betty Berzon's *Permanent Partners*, Rik Isensee's *Love between Men*, Tina Tessina's *Gay Relationships*, John Driggs and Steve Finn's *Intimacy Between Men*, and Merilee Clunis and Dorsey Green's *Lesbian Couples*.

But the biggest development has been the interest in matters spiritual. Dennis Paddie, an Austin poet and playwright working to bring spiritual perspectives on AIDS into the mainstream, has commented in conversation with me that he does not know of any relatively conscious gay man who has *not* been compelled in the face of AIDS to develop some sort of theological or metaphysical explanation. It seems almost axiomatic (perhaps because it is tautological?) that facing death forces human beings to step outside the concerns of daily life and ask transcendent questions about the nature and meaning of life. Within gay and, to a slightly less urgent degree, lesbian cultures new spiritualities are being born.

Thus another growing subgenre is the gay/lesbian spiritual book: for example, Arthur Evans' *Witchcraft and the Gay Counterculture*, to cite the classic in this area; also Walter Williams's *The Spirit and the Flesh*, Judy Grahn's *Another Mother Tongue*, Mark Thompson's anthology *Gay Spirit: Myth and Meaning*, Roger Lanphear's *Gay Spirituality*, J. Michael Clark's *A Place to Start*, Sonia Johnson's *Going Out of Our Minds*, and, in the current-day manifestation of pseudepigraphal prophecy (i.e., "trance-channeling") Andrew Ramer's *Two Flutes Playing.*

In the same way that gay tastes are often in the vanguard in art, style, and culture, emerging gay spiritualities probably hint at the future direction of human spiritual consciousness in general. And, for the most part, these inchoately developing spiritualities are nature-centered, ecological, egalitarian, evolutionary-based, secular, and post-Christian (in the sense that they generally embrace the teachings of Jesus Christ while dismissing the Christian religion that seems to have long since abandoned the loving and nonjudgmental, anti-institutional and nonlegalistic attitude Jesus taught and for which he himself was executed by the religious establishment of his own day). The gay experience of AIDS as a call to spiritual consciousness and compassion is a step toward reclaiming the spiritual identity as shamans and witch doctors, faeries and oracles—mystical leaders—that gay historical and anthropological research reveal male and female homosexuals and cross-dressers have had in other cultures and other times.

Why would homosexual orientation produce vanguard spiritual intuitions? one might legitimately ask. The answer is twofold. First, by its very nature spiritual intuition stands outside mainstream assumptions and values to achieve a perspective in which nonobvious associations can be made that link diverse elements of experience, creating what we generally call "meaning." And, by *their* very nature, it seems, homosexual men and women live outside the mainstream assumptions and values.

As children, lesbians and gay men sense that "we don't belong," "we aren't wanted (as gay)," "we are different," "we are outsiders." The ecclesiastical gay spiritual writer and Episcopalian priest John Fortunato calls this an experience of being "exiles." The secular gay spiritual writer and editor Paul Reed calls it "longing." In *Serenity,* Reed writes eloquently of an experience that is "integral to those of us who have been spiritually deprived by a society which denies us the food for our souls and hearts" (11–13):

> Gay people are groomed for longing by the very fact of the lack of a place for gay people within society. . . . We are kind and gentle people. We are a loving community from which violence does not readily erupt. But it is this difference of spirit—this kindness of spirit—that also feeds longing, for the schism between this loving mode of our community and the rough mode of a world we want to remake can be profound. We wish that things were different; we long for them to be otherwise, on a spiritual as well as physical plane, just as we longed for different surroundings and attitudes as gay children and teenagers coping hopelessly in a foreign land.

... surely the world is filled with loving nongays who, too, long for social change (though I have always wondered about a certain question here—do we seek social change and spiritual serenity because we are gay, or are we gay because we seek social and spiritual change?). (11–13)

In a sometimes harrowing, sometimes devastating, almost always heroic way, recognizing homosexual orientation forces individuals to reassess their place in society and often, in the process, to question societal assumptions. Gay men and lesbians are forced by socially sanctioned homophobia to achieve some kind of critical distance from which they can find their own experience included in the experience of being human. Indeed, if there is such a thing as a gay sensibility, it probably derives from individuals being forced by their aberrant sexuality into critical stance on life in general.

Gay people learn to be observers rather than participants. That sense of being excluded may ironically be the source of most of their sufferings (low self-esteem, dissatisfaction, sexual restlessness, compulsivity, etc.) as well as of their specialness (sensitivity, awareness, compassion, artisticness, taste, etc.). Indeed, it may be that, irrespective of the hostility of the scribes and pharisees[1] of the modern-day Church, it is this sense of being outside and wanting more that leaves gay people dissatisfied with conventional religion.

Second, this forced perception from critical distance puts gay people in the vanguard because it is not only an *aspect* of spiritual experience but the *hallmark* of contemporary experience in general and postmodern consciousness in particular. For critical distance from the beliefs and assumptions of specific cultures is precisely the consequence the human race is being forced into by modern technology and worldwide communication. Changes in the world in the last hundred years (easy travel, mass communication, financial interdependence, exposure to the variety of human cultures, technological achievement) have forced all people to perceive the world from beyond their own culture.

The world religionist Joseph Campbell has observed that the potent spiritual/mythic image of today is the view of Earth seen from the Moon. For the first time in history, human beings have been able to achieve a perspective from which to view the whole of the human universe. Campbell notes that this parallels the psychological experience of viewing one's self and one's culture from over and above. And this changes everything. No longer can a person imagine his or her beliefs and opinions to be obvious and universal. No longer can any one culture claim its "truth" to be superior. No longer can any people actually believe (except out of reactionary defensiveness and insecurity) that their god is the only true god, their precious savior the only savior, and that the millions of other human beings who worship differently are totally deluded.

The stance of being outside and above the content of individual religions forces one into a kind of Buddhistic metareligion in which it is not the content of religion but the fact of religious questing that provides inspiration and enlightenment. Gay people are naturals for such metareligion, for by their gayness they are propelled willy-nilly into that perspective. Not all survive and thrive, just as not all people appreciate the new vision of humanity revealed by the lunar perspective. But gay culture incorporates this higher perspective, witnessing to it by the essence of gay sexuality—if not always by the actual behavior of gay and lesbian people.

This metareligion effects a kind of detachment from the details of day-to-day life, perhaps because it suggests that there are not facile, obvious answers to the significant transcendent questions—that is, it inculcates a critical stance on the questions themselves. Such pure forms of spirituality urge virtues of detachment, patience, and compassion, reminding the individual that he or she is more than just the body, more than just the daily routine, more than just the physical and emotional suffering. Of its very essence, spirituality is about life in a larger, more expanded context, beyond the immediacy of time and space, beyond the demands of ego.

It probably doesn't matter whether such an expanded, ego-transcending viewpoint is "really true"—for example, whether human beings have souls or whether we reincarnate or are part of God. What matters is that achieving a critical stance on ego and on the problems of day-to-day living frees one from the problems and questions and allows a kind of joy, even in the face of suffering. This joy comes from experiencing meaning, and meaning comes from experiencing things in a larger context.

As at other critical times in human history—and as we are facing the turn of the millennium and the turn of the age—we are discovering larger contexts and experiencing major paradigm shifts. The models of the world and of our human experience are changing, which we sense as a dramatic change in what is thought to be true.

Science—the language human beings currently use to interpret experience—has undermined the religious revelations of ages past. Evangelical fundamentalism has been enjoying a hey-day in the 1980s, yet scientific realism has won the battle over which institutions in society establish truth. Doubtless, in a hundred years or less a new paradigm of reality will supplant the materialism of twentieth-century science. In all likelihood—given the direction science has been going in the latter half of the century—the new paradigm(s) will incorporate human consciousness into scientific materialism or, conversely, incorporate the material world into the larger reality of consciousness, understanding the physical world as a projection onto three-dimensional space of a higher multidimensional reality that includes what we now call "spirit."

Such a paradigm shift will be mediated by laboratory findings and philosophical dissertations and by cultural upheavals and social disasters and triumphs. The contention of this essay is that the rise of a gay counterculture in the 1970s in the dominant Western society and its battle with the tragedy of AIDS in the 1980s play an integral—and even leading—role in the development of new paradigms of human nature, especially in the area of spirituality.

One basis of this contention is that in a world about to be devastated by runaway population growth, condoning and even encouraging a stable percentage of homosexuals may be ecologically adaptive. As society is further debilitated by the collapse of child-rearing institutions and the breakup of the family, it only makes sense to encourage people with psychological tendencies that might work against their forming strong and nurturing traditional families—from certain styles of homosexual orientation to a history of sexual or emotional victimization—to eschew marrying and reproducing. (Why pressure repressed homosexuals, for instance, into marrying and having children in their twenties only to have them finally acknowledge their sexuality and break up their families in their thirties? Yet this is a major strategy of the fundamentalists who are trying to "save the family." Isn't it obvious that the people who should be parents are those who have sex because they want children and not those who have children because they want sex?) Gay consciousness points the way toward reestablishing priorities in human life that justify and reinforce population reduction and concern about the quality of life over the expansion of population.

In the wide view of history this may be appropriately symmetrical. The studies of the Yale classics scholar John Boswell have revealed that homosexual activity only came to be universally condemned in the Christian West in the fourteenth century, during the time of the devastation of the Hundred Years War and the Black Death. An implication to be drawn from his research is that, at least for reasons of organizational maintenance, the Church needed to encourage repopulation and to explain how its omnipotent God could have allowed these disasters. Condemning nonprocreative sex accomplished both in one swoop: homosexuals were scapegoated with the disaster and the populace was intimidated into reproductive heterosexuality. Boswell's research shows that after that time biblical passages—the story of Sodom and Gomorrah among them—that had not previously been so interpreted were then given antihomosexual interpretations.

For modern homosexuals that reinterpretation of scripture has proved disastrous—even the United States Supreme Court considered it a precedent to permit states to deny civil rights protections to homosexual citizens. In the Middle Ages, however, it was at least better than the Church's previous attempt to explain the plague by blaming witches—for the subsequent slaughter of cats, believed to be witches' familiars, eliminated the most important predator of the rats that we now know were the carriers of the real vector for the bubonic plague. Blaming the homosexuals didn't worsen that epidemic; blaming the cats did. In contemporary times, on the other hand, blaming homosexuals for the epidemic of AIDS—perhaps out of the same kind of Church organizational maintenance and aggrandizement concerns and superstitions—has worsened the epidemic by delaying public health interventions, discrediting early research, and—even a decade into the epidemic—confusing education about how HIV is spread.

Ironically, AIDS may be the undoing of the superstitions spawned by the Black Death, for in the twentieth century, the incidence of this new epidemic has again affected how sexuality and homosexuality are perceived. For all that AIDS has been a tragedy and a setback for civil rights–organizing efforts, it has also squarely established the existence and identity of a gay subculture, made "gay" a household word, and encouraged and legitimated intellectual investigation of alternative sexualities.

And for a variety of reasons—some validated, some debunked by Susan Sontag's discussions of illness as metaphor—AIDS has sparked new awareness of the role of consciousness in the functioning of the body. In ways that are both hokey, even quackish, as well as solidly scientific, AIDS has generated such disciplines as psycho-neuro-immunology and brought attention to such previously esoteric notions as creative visualization, self-fulfilling prophecy, and energy flow in the body-mind-person. In the 1990s, the concerns of spirituality tend to be energy flow (which in meditation and prayer can be brought into awareness), the interconnection of these energies with other persons and with the Earth itself, and the power of thought to create the future. The old Cartesian notion that the body is a machine controlled by the mind is fading and with it the mechanistic notion that bodies and minds are individuated and cut off from one another.

The paradigm shift that is happening today—and that gay people are inchoately leading—is that, with critical perspective, we can now see the process. We understand the myths not as depictions of reality but as metaphors available to us for figuring out how to relate to that part of ourselves that is creating our experience and generating the influences that we have in the world around us.

This metareligious model changes the notion of God. The relationship and interaction human beings have with God is perhaps like the relationships we have with animals, that is, with beings on the other end of the continuum of consciousness and intelligence. In the same way that we imagine a personality in our cat, so we imagine—and project onto—a personality in God. But when we're talking to our cat, we're really talking to ourselves about the quality of our experience of having the cat. We enjoy talking to our animals and imagining they have personalities just like us; we name them and seek to divine traits in their behavior that reveal our influence on them (e.g., what we've taught them, what they do for love of us). Similarly, when we're speaking with God we're really talking to ourselves about the quality of our experience of being alive and conscious. The proper effort in life, that is, to love God, is to enhance that experience, to make life richer and fuller, and to have influence on the world around us which makes the experience of others richer and fuller.

That part of ourselves that we are talking to when we talk to God is a powerful force in the creation of our experience. In some ways we can't understand from this level of consciousness, simply because here we're individual egoistic beings seemingly out of touch with the other levels, part of each of us is the Creator of the universe of experience in which each of us lives and interacts with others. The myths come down to us as suggestions for how we can imagine the personality of God so that we can relate properly to that part of ourselves.

Just as the cat is really there, so God is really there. But what God is can only be experienced by symbols and metaphors. This discovery changes the way we relate to those symbols and metaphors. We see that we don't have to accept the ones that have been used in the past, that we can edit the myths we have inherited, that we can reshape them by observing the similarities and differences and by observing the influence they have in the world around us. For instance, metaphors for God which result in war and racism can be understood today to be maladaptive. And we can stop talking about God like that.

In fact, we have to. That's the moral obligation of the coming times: to re-create God, which is to say, to construct the phenomenon of God appropriate for our present reality.

A consequence of the modern ability to view the world from a global perspective is the awareness of natural ecology. We see that different cultures, religions, and belief systems developed historically in response to practical problems. Indeed, we can begin to see that the growth of life on Earth represents some sort of evolution of a planetary, collective being—called, in New Age mythology, Gaia.

Perhaps our planet itself is an organized and unified organism, not unlike our own bodies, that grows according to instructions contained in something we could call "etheric DNA" (the evolutionary biologist Rupert Sheldrake might call this "the morphogenetic fields" [*Rebirth* 97ff.]). Just as our bodies grow and change without our conscious intention—or particular attention to the instructions—so Earth grows and changes according to the observable dynamics of ecology and the rules of evolution. Earth may not consciously design specific coded communication, but nonetheless it may be communicating with us through our history just as the secretions in our bodies communicate with our cells.

Gaia necessarily communicates through sexuality (sex being the dynamic of evolution as it is experienced by individual human beings). And so the development of identified gay cultures and gay consciousness ought to be seen (i.e., mythologized) as a message from Gaia.

Concern with these communications has generally been called spirituality. The function of spirituality is to explain—in myth and symbol understandable to human beings—what is going on at a higher, global, metalevel, that is, what Gaia is trying to tell us. AIDS is surely one of those practical problems that shape the direction of human consciousness. AIDS has to be mythologized and explained in ways that provide positive messages about Earth's ecology. AIDS, after all, is one of the first truly major ecodisasters of modern urbanity, and the gay community's collective response has been—at least in most instances—exemplary of the kind of grassroots organizing and community mobilization for problem solving that will be demanded more and more in the future.

The struggle of spiritually concerned individuals is to figure out what the lesson is that AIDS conveys from Gaia—or, in other words, to place AIDS in the context of the larger evolution of the planet. The interpretation we construct for AIDS along the road of trials must explain our experience for ourselves in a way that makes our lives better and makes us influence other lives around us for the better. If nothing else, AIDS has revealed gay compassion and given the world an example to follow.

For almost 10 percent of the population, the 1980s were characterized by a plague that, seemingly out of nowhere, swept through their lives, cutting down friends and lovers and threatening to lurk secretly in their own bloodstreams. And while gay men watched their brothers die mysteriously, society didn't seem to care. Doctors didn't want to treat the disease. Ministers blamed it on the victims. The Church actively fought strategies to curtail the spread. The president of the United States couldn't even bring himself to say "AIDS."

In the face of this indifference and hostility, gay men and lesbians joined together to assist the sick and dying. Gay community groups across the country organized buddy programs, psychological support groups, bereavement workshops, safe-sex training classes—all to ease the pain and stop the virus. Women and men came forward to visit and help people with AIDS—people who were often strangers to them, who had a disease other Americans were so frightened of they wanted all the sufferers locked away in quarantine. The volunteers fed and cleaned up after the PWAs; they helped them bathe; they emptied their bedpans. And they did this not for a few days when it was in vogue and the focus of a super rock concert but for months and even years. In spite of enormous opposition from mainstream society, lesbians and gay men cared for one another and virtually stemmed the spread of the virus in their own communities. Such caring was born not out of guilt or fear of divine wrath but out of compassion.

In *AIDS: A Passageway to Transformation,* Norman Shealy and Caroline Myss argue that one message of AIDS is that "victim consciousness"— that is, the experience of being powerless in face of intolerable experience—is literally killing the human race (38). Metaphorically, AIDS manifests victimhood and defenselessness—that, indeed, is precisely what the virus causes. By responding with compassion, gay men and lesbians have demonstrated the proper cure for victimhood. As a world, we must learn compassion. And we must learn compassion for the world, not just for other human beings.

Gay people are the saints—offering their bodies for medical experimentation to save maybe themselves but certainly future generations. And they manifest that saints can be liberated and even libertine so long as they are compassionate and do not cause harm to others. In that they are manifesting the significant teachings of the world saviors of the past. And they are recovering our ancient spiritual roles as eccentrics, shamans, prophets, and mystical beings. The moral and spiritual imperative for gay men and lesbians is to recognize these changes in their status and reshape their lives; for non-gay men and women it is to rethink their notions of sexuality according to a new paradigm.

The gay plight manifests a whole new vision of how society should operate, with efforts turned to helping the misfortunate instead of blaming them. The gay response to AIDS reveals something crucial about the way to envision the rules of reality on the next level up (i.e., how to envision the personality of God) and that is that nobody is wrong, that we can help people without blaming anybody, that we can solve the problems in society without having to make some people wrong so other people can be right. In other words, we can learn to forgive and to discover that in forgiveness comes healing.

One manifestation of the process of creation—which is usually posed not in spiritual but in philosophical and sociological terms—is the so-called essentialist/constructionist debate raging in gay and lesbian intellectual circles. The debate, which originated in the thought of the French philosopher and martyr to AIDS Michel Foucault, centers on the question of whether homosexual orientation is a result of inherent, essential biological factors that have remained relatively constant throughout human history (like left-handedness, for instance) or a result of sociological influences that have ebbed and flowed in different ways in different times and cultures and produced different kinds of homosexualities. (In ancient times, for instance, homosexual acts seemed to be linked to domination and violence—even in Greece, where the violence was quelled by civilization, but the domination-submission was not. The oft-touted prohibition in Leviticus was more likely a condemnation of the male dominance practice of anally raping one's enemies after victory in battle than a condemnation of same-sex expression of affection between equals.)

A less felicitous version applies these questions to personality development, recapitulating the nature versus nurture debate in psychology and raising the consequent question of whether homosexuality can be changed. In conversation with me, Peter Goldblum, co-author with Martin Delaney of *Strategies for Survival*, observed that in individual development only an "interactionist" model makes sense: the developing person feels preverbal sexual urgings and then learns to name them according to the socially—and sociologically—constructed terms and norms of his or her time and place.

Because the debate is generally posed in scientific terms, the proofs and disproofs are sought in historical evidence. A spiritual approach to the debate might offer other insights by pointing out that both biological essence and social construction are themselves constructed in consciousness and may be best understood as messages from Gaia. In that sense, homosexuality as we know it today (as gay consciousness) may be a relatively recent phenomenon created by karmic, morphogenetic influences on the evolution of the Earth.

The evolutionary mystic Teilhard de Chardin said humankind is evolution become conscious and responsible for its direction (133–38). Gay men and lesbians may have a special role to play in the construction of new metaphors of human life, in part simply because they manifest the phenomenon of construction. This is the most important message of the essentialist/constructionist debate: by discussing it, we are modifying our understanding of ourselves; we are engaged in "revolution through consciousness change."

Part of that revolution may be a discovery about the nature of sex—namely, its psychoneurological and evolutionary function. This notion comes out of bodywork psychology and Eastern meditation. Wilhelm Reich, one of Freud's more unusual disciples, observed that orgasm floods the nervous system with energy that in some way has the potential for healing the psyche. Reich hypothesized that neurosis—and indirectly cancer—was a result of constrictions in the flow of psychic energy in the brain and body. A fully experienced orgasm, he believed, flushed the nervous system of the constrictions and so brought psychological health (Kramer).

With the possible exception of cetaceans, human beings are the only animals that don't have sex out of instinct or hormonal and pheromonal drives. (Apparently, some people do, but as a race we've evolved beyond that.) Our sexual patterns are different from all other animals: our females are continuously—rather than cyclically—available and experience specific female orgasm in intercourse (which is not essential for reproduction and therefore not necessarily a trait created by natural selection, which seems concerned only with reproduction). And we engage in expressions of affection and elaborate genital stimulation in foreplay which generate an altered state of consciousness. (As the spiritual erotic massage therapist Joseph Kramer points out, this consciousness is parallel to that sought in Tantric Yoga through the raising of the Kundalini, which is the divine creative energy that vivifies the body and generates the experience of the mind.)

The other thing, of course, that is different about us is that we've evolved intelligence—which is also a state of consciousness. Perhaps evolving the sexual patterns we did resulted in the kind of orgasms we have, which in turn created the brain mechanisms that spawn intelligence. Perhaps, for instance, the psychic flushing stimulated the growth of brain cells and consciousness.

Today, one role of homosexuals in the evolution of consciousness on Earth may be to manifest and facilitate the realization that sex has other functions besides reproduction, that is, to identify the role of sex as psychological experience, worthwhile for its own sake. Indeed, the altered state of consciousness of sexual arousal, especially between consenting equals, free of violence, dominance, or greed, is beneficent. An aligned function may be to act as midwife for the evolutionary transformation. Some of the traits of gay people that blend masculinity and femininity result in personalities that are amazingly creative and sensitive and nurturing, and these guide the development of humanness. Of course, there are many homosexuals who don't fit this model of visionaries and creators of the future, just as there are many heterosexuals who don't fit the model of good procreators and parents of the next generation.

This role for homosexuals is relatively new. Only recently have conscious lesbians and gay men, as we know them, appeared—people who blend gender traits and whose sole interest in sex is to form relationship for intimacy and relationships' sake, not because of any biological necessity. This moves the whole system up a notch into spiritual evolution.

The paradigm shift in the experience of sexuality—which is the spiritual message of gay love—is that we can and should love creation, emotionally and physically, for its own sake. We must love the world as it is. We must love beauty in the material world and strive to enhance it. We must save the physical Earth. We must love life, love experience, and seek richness of experience and find in that experience the manifestation of God.

This is a radical overturning of traditional religious myths, which taught that salvation was always in the future, that is, beyond the grave and not on this physical planet, and that an individual's function was to obey rules and to be useful, to contribute to population growth—and the wealth of his or her own culture in competition with other cultures—and to assist dominant males in propagating their genes into the future (where salvation lay). This was an intensely egoistic system. It was useful for populating and conquering a world often hostile and threatening to human beings. Now, however, it is human beings who are hostile and threatening to the world. And the propagation of specific genes is now no longer as important as the construction of a society that honors Earth and seeks to create beauty and harmony. With Earth so full, the struggle for genetic continuation (i.e., immortality through offspring) by dominant males is no longer adaptive. This is the message of feminism. And the gay contribution to this radical overturning of past models is sensitivity to beauty for its own sake.

Ironically, the fundamentalists object to homosexuality as "fruitless" and "selfish." In fact, the fruit that gay men and lesbians produce in the world is not just propagation of themselves but expressions of beauty (God's beauty) for all to share. This is far less selfish than overcrowding the world with children for the sake of preserving males' genes—as though we still needed more. And from this gay contribution flows a morality that makes sense today—when moral laws from old books no longer do. For if we love life and seek to enhance our own experience and the experience of others in a crowded world, then we *are* compassionate, and from that, *properly,* flows all morality.

Politicized feminist-identified lesbians and, to a less imprisoning degree, gay-identified men often impose upon themselves a standard of political correctness that demands they embrace every cause and movement they become aware of for social justice and against oppression. This political correctness can be at least as disciplining as the sex-confining morality of Christianity, but more useful. In general, lesbians and gay men seem to have more liberal attitudes about sex and drugs than the mainstream populace—because they see that these are really issues of social control (concerned with abstract principles), not of virtue and morality—while they are much more concerned about issues of fairness and kindness (concerned with persons).

In that regard, feminism and gay liberation dramatically manifest the real teachings of spiritual religion. We have faced the edge of history and seen how the human race can save itself. And the announcement of this teaching is the boon of our hero's journey born from ordeal along the road of trials.

Note

1. These technical terms of turn-of-the-era Hebrew religion are properly translated "Church officials and conservative religious leaders." Even two thousand years ago Jesus knew religious wisdom shouldn't be left in the hands of the Church.

Works Cited

Barrus, Tim. *Genocide: The Anthology.* Stamford, Conn.: Knights Press, 1989.

Berzon, Betty. *Permanent Partners: Building Gay and Lesbian Relationships That Last.* New York: New American Library, 1989.

Boswell, John. *Christianity, Social Tolerance and Homosexuality.* Chicago: University of Chicago Press, 1980.

Campbell, Joseph. *The Hero with a Thousand Faces.* Princeton, N.J.: Princeton University Press, 1954.

Clark, Don. *The New Loving Someone Gay.* Berkeley: Celestial Arts, 1987.

Clark, J. Michael. *A Place to Start.* Dallas: Monument Press, 1989.

Clunis, Merilee, and Dorsey Green. *Lesbian Couples.* Seattle: Seal Press, 1988.

Cooper, Dennis. *Closer.* New York: Grove, 1989.

Driggs, John, and Stephen Finn. *Intimacy Between Men.* New York: New American Library, 1989.

Evans, Arthur. *Witchcraft and the Gay Counterculture.* Boston: Fag Rag, 1978.

Feinberg, David. *Eighty-sixed.* New York: Penguin, 1989.

Ferro, Robert. *Second Son.* New York: New American Library, 1988.

Forster, E. M. *Maurice.* New York: Norton, 1971.

Fortunato, John. *Embracing the Exile.* San Francisco: Seabury, 1982.

Goldblum, Peter, and Martin Delaney. *Strategies for Survival.* New York: St. Martin's Press, 1987.

Grahn, Judy. *Another Mother Tongue.* Boston: Beacon, 1984.

Greenberg, David. *The Construction of Homosexuality.* Chicago: University of Chicago Press, 1988.

Hay, Louise. *The AIDS Book: Creating a Positive Approach.* Los Angeles: Hay House, 1988.

Isensee, Rik. *Love between Men.* New York: Prentice Hall, 1990.

Johnson, Sonia. *Going Out of Our Minds.* Watsonville, Calif.: Crossing Press, 1988.

Johnson, Edwin Clark (Toby). *Secret Matter.* South Norwalk, Conn.: Lavender Press, 1990.

Kramer, Joseph. *Ecstatic Sex, Healthy Sex.* Audio tape. Oakland: Body Electric Publishing, 1988.

Lanphear, Roger. *Gay Spirituality.* San Diego: Unified Publications, 1990.

Marotta, Toby. *The Politics of Homosexuality.* Boston: Houghton-Mifflin, 1981.

Monette, Paul. *Borrowed Time.* San Diego: Harcourt, Brace, Jovanovich, 1988.

———. *Afterlife.* New York: Crown, 1990.

Ramer, Andrew. *Two Flutes Playing.* Oakland: Body Electric Publishing, 1987.

Reed, Paul. *Serenity.* 2d ed. Berkeley: Celestial Arts, 1990.

Reich, Charles. *The Greening of America.* New York: Bantam Books, 1971.

Roszak, Theodore. *The Making of a Counter-culture.* New York: Doubleday, 1972.

Shealy, Norman, and Caroline Myss. *AIDS: A Passageway to Transformation.* Walpole, N.H.: Stillpoint, 1989.

Sheldrake, Rupert. *The Rebirth of Nature: The Greening of Science and God.* New York: Bantam Books, 1991.

Sontag, Susan. *AIDS and Its Metaphors.* New York: Farrar, Straus, Giroux, 1989.

Teilhard de Chardin, Pierre. *The Divine Milieu.* New York: Harper and Row, 1960.

Tessina, Tina. *Gay Relationships.* Los Angeles: Tarcher, 1989.

Thompson, Mark, ed. *Gay Spirit: Myth and Meaning.* New York: St. Martin's Press, 1987.

Warren, Patricia Nell. *The Front Runner.* New York: New American Library, 1974.

Weinrich, James. *Sexual Landscapes.* New York: Macmillan, 1987.

Williams, Walter. *The Spirit and the Flesh.* Boston: Beacon, 1986.

PART TWO

Literary AIDS:
A Sampling

The Very Same

From *Love Alone: 18 Elegies for Rog*

the wrongest of the wrong things said that day
as I stepped from the chapel an idiot cousin
once-removed jiggled my shoulder *time to turn
the page* intoned like it's all been so appalling
we must hasten now to the land of brunch
there to recover our BMWs our zest for
winning and half-acre closets sorry I'm
booked weeks later still fuming with retorts
BUT THIS IS MY PAGE IT CANNOT BE TURNED
then start hearing similar from other bimbos
gotta turn the page Paul is this shit from
the Bible the sayings of Dr. Kubler-Ross
has Donohue done a show on it maybe
a ring of widows all walks of life neatly
combining real estate aerobics and young
blue-collar bowling dates spare me the pop
coping skills this page is all that's left of time
there *was* no page before I caught you the book
was nothing but cover painfully thin and
hopelessly derivative there's something French
in all of this perhaps *la vie continue*
well no it doesn't not if you freeze it in its
tracks think of this turnless page like Audubon's
elephant folio where the eagle is life-size
or a gilded Burgundian leaf of hours painted
with a one-hair brush for the whole last half
of the 1400s and no bigger than a 3 × 5
dear friend I didn't become your blood brother
lightly mine ticks just like yours but a beat

slower the Geiger of Death crackles in every
room yet He cannot seem to tell who's who
as you used to say in your cranked-up bed
playful astonished *But we're the same person
when did that happen* with Death's signals jammed
I and my page have eluded the dart awhile
Russians in bughouses write their poems on soap
with burnt matches then get them by heart then
wash in muddy water think what they would do
with a whole page no room left on ours edge
to edge with our growing interchangeability
what you would do I think is make a paper
glider go to the brink of a high green place
let it cavort the updrafts lulling itself
by lightness to the valley floor below
while I am more likely to paper the walls
with mine scrawling *why* and *where are you*
in our common blood how shall we compromise
would a kite do do you think riding its string
in the upper air and don't forget there's
an eagle on it and the monk's gilt borders
my blood cries are too high up to read now
oh what a page Rog how can they not see
I am only still here to be with you
my best my only page scribbled on cirrus
the high air soaring in its every word

AIDS

From *The Silence Now: New and Collected Earlier Poems*

We are stretched to meet a new dimension
Of love, a more demanding range
Where despair and hope must intertwine.
How grow to meet it? Intention
Here can neither move nor change
The raw truth. Death is on the line.
It comes to separate and estrange
Lover from lover in some reckless design.
Where do we go from here?

Fear. Fear. Fear. Fear.

Our world has never been more stark
Or more in peril.
It is very lonely now in the dark.
Lonely and sterile.

And yet in the simple turn of a head
Mercy lives. I heard it when someone said
"I must go now to a dying friend.
Every night at nine I tuck him into bed,
And give him a shot of morphine,"
And added, "I go where I have never been."
I saw he meant into a new discipline
He had not imagined before, and a new grace.

Every day now we meet it face to face.
Every day now devotion is the test.
Through the long hours, the hard, caring nights
We are forging a new union. We are blest.

As closed hands open to each other
Closed lives open to strange tenderness.
We are learning the hard way how to mother.
Who says it is easy? But we have the power.
I watch the faces deepen all around me.
It is the time of change, the saving hour.
The word suddenly made new,
As we learn it again, as we bring it alive:

Love. Love. Love. Love.

Aunt Ida Pieces a Quilt

You are right, but your patch isn't big enough.
—Jesse Jackson

When a cure is found and the last panel is sewn into
place, the Quilt will be displayed in a permanent
home as a national monument to the individual, irre-
placeable people lost to AIDS—and the people who
knew and loved them most.
—Cleve Jones, founder, The NAMES Project

They brought me some of his clothes. The hospital gown,
those too-tight dungarees, his blue choir robe
with the gold sash. How that boy could sing!
His favorite color in a necktie. A Sunday shirt.
What I'm gonna do with all this stuff?
I can remember Junie without this business.
My niece Francine say they quilting all over the country.
So many good boys like her boy, gone.

At my age I ain't studying no needle and thread.
My eyes ain't so good now and my fingers lock in a fist,
they so eaten up with arthritis. This old back
don't take kindly to bending over a frame no more.
Francine say ain't I a mess carrying on like this.
I could make two quilts the time I spend running my mouth.

Just cut his name out the cloths, stitch something nice
about him. Something to bring him back. You can do it,
Francine say. Best sewing our family ever had.
Quilting ain't that easy, I say. Never was easy.
Y'all got to help me remember him good.

Most of my quilts was made down South. My mama
and my mama's mama taught me. Popped me on the tail
if I missed a stich or threw the pattern out of line.
I did "Bright Star" and "Lonesome Square" and "Rally Round,"
what many folks don't bother with nowadays. Then Elmo and me
married and came North where the cold in Connecticut
cuts you like a knife. We was warm, though.
We had sackcloth and calico and cotton, 100% pure.
What they got now but polyester rayon. Factory made.

Let me tell you something. In all my quilts there's a secret
nobody knows. Every last one of them got my name Ida
stitched on the back side in red thread.
That's where Junie got his flair. Don't let nobody fool you.
When he got the youth choir standing up and singing
the whole church would rock. He'd throw up his hands
from them wide blue sleeves and the church would hush
right down to the funeral parlor fans whisking the air.
He'd toss his head back and holler and we'd all cry holy.

And never mind his too-tight dungarees.
I caught him switching down the street one Saturday night,
and I seen him more than once. I said, Junie,
you ain't got to let the world know all your business.
Who cared where he went when he wanted to have fun.
He'd be singing his heart out come Sunday morning.

When Francine say she gonna hang this quilt in the church
I like to fall out. A quilt ain't no showpiece,
it's to keep you warm. Francine say it can do both.
Now I ain't so old-fashioned I can't change,
but I made Francine come over and bring her daughter
Belinda. We cut and tacked his name, JUNIE.
Just plain and simple. "JUNIE, *our boy.*"
Cut the J in blue, the U in gold. N in dungarees
just as tight as you please. The I from the hospital gown
and the white shirt he wore First Sunday. Belinda
put the necktie E in the cross-stitch I showed her.

Wouldn't you know we got to talking about Junie.
We could smell him in the cloth.
Underarm. Afro Sheen pomade. Gravy stains.
I forgot all about my arthritis.
When Francine left me to finish up, I swear

I heard Junie giggling right along with me
as I stitched IDA on the back side in red thread.

Francine say she gonna send this quilt to Washington
like folks doing from all 'cross the country,
so many good people gone. Babies, mothers, fathers
and boys like our Junie. Francine say
they gonna piece this quilt to another one,
another name and another patch
all in a larger quilt getting larger and larger.

Maybe we all like that, patches waiting to be pieced.
Well, I don't know about Washington
We need Junie here with us. And Maxine,
she cousin May's husband's sister's people,
she having a baby and here comes winter already.
The cold cutting like knives. Now where did I put that needle?

Note

Melvin Dixon died of AIDS on October 26, 1992, while this book was in production.

Voices

"They're calling it the 'Gay Plague.'"
"Pleasure is death."
"Danger is half the fun."
"They're getting their just desserts."
"We're already exposed. Why fight it?"
"It's just another Damocles' Sword. We've always had them."
"It's God's punishment."
"Don't tell me any more. I don't want to know."
"Why should I worry?"
"So what's changed? It's us against them."
"The Angel of Death will pass over us."
"Maybe it will mutate to a harmless form."
"We're dropping like flies."
"Geometric progression."
"If you've got it, you deserve it."
"They're out to get us, one way or another."
"I hear it's germ warfare. Tested it on fags. Double benefit."
"Pure paranoia."
"One hundred percent mortality rate."
"You gotta die sometime."
"We're all going to die."
"Well, I'm going to enjoy myself while I can."
"What have I done to deserve this?"
"Get 'em while they're down."
"It's nature getting rid of its mistakes."
"What's the use of trying?"
"We can lick this if we all pull together."
"Look what you've done to us and our children!"
"Hope springs eternal."
"Somebody's got to speak up."
"Just another freak crying wolf."

"A voice crying in the wilderness."

"Repent!"

"Science can cure anything."

"Money's the answer."

"There are no atheists in foxholes."

"God is dead."

"If it were someone else, they'd try harder."

"There may be no tomorrow, but I'm available tonight."

"Good riddance."

"Wait until it crosses over to the general population."

"If no one else will help, we'll help ourselves."

"Disease equals guilt."

"Don't tell anyone, please. It would kill my mother if she knew."

"Naturally, you can't go on working. It would cause a panic."

"Hope you've got good insurance."

"We'll get along, somehow."

"And he threw you out?"

"Of course, they *said* it was cancer."

"A rogue by any other name . . . "

"AIDS, huh? So he's a faggot. Always thought so."

"How could a priest get it?"

"Serves 'em right. Fags, druggies, and whores."

"They're infecting the innocents: children, hemophiliacs, surgical
    patients."

"We're twentieth-century plague rats. You know, vermin bearing vermin."

"Guilt by association."

"Relative guilt, selective condemnation."

"PWAs. The new pariahs."

"Yes, he's coming out the hard way."

"God will protect me."

"I was born lucky."

"It's roulette, nothing more."

"Rubbers? You can't feel a thing."

"It's their disease."

"Women don't get it."

"Never had anal sex, I swear."

"Never had oral sex, I swear."

"How far can I go without catching it?"

"Sure, and the leopard's gonna change his spots."

"Quarantine them."

"Better still, kill them before they kill us."

"He just retreated into himself and never came out."

"Why me, Lord?"

"Good people don't get it."

"Good people only get it by accident."

"God, good people are getting it. See what they started?"

"It's pure malice. They're trying to drag us all down with them."

"He was so young. Tragic."

"Oh well, he'd lived his life anyway."

"If you repent, maybe God will change His mind."

"Repent and at least die with dignity and a clean conscience."

"Maybe there will be a miracle."

"No miracle in my case, anyway."

"There are no miracles."

"It's only a disease, for God's sake."

"Stay out of it. It's not our problem."

"Tested? Hell no, you think I want everybody in the world to know I'm
     gay?"

"They know more than they're telling us."

"They're waiting until production becomes profitable."

"They're dragging their feet because of who is dying."

"They're doing the best they can with what they have to work with."

"Human guinea pigs. That's all we are."

"If I'm going down, I'm going down fighting."

"They are letting this go on, wanting it to go on."

"This is political dynamite—or suicide. Don't get involved."

"Promise anything, but do nothing."

"AIDS should be the nation's number one priority."

"There's a fortune to be made here."

"It's snake oil time again."

"I'll do anything."

"Somebody's got to have the answer."

"There's no one so gullible as the desperate."

"Separation of wheat from chaff. No more. Not worth your effort or
     sympathy."

"Trust no one."

"You've got to trust someone, believe in something. Without that you're
     dead before you die."

"If I can just hang on a little longer, there's bound to be a breakthrough."

"I've cried until I'm hollow."

"You know, of course, he wasn't there when they displayed the quilt."

"So much love. Why does it take death to bring out love?"

"The family threw his lover out."

"His own mother wouldn't see him."

"It was the only time in their lives they were that close."

"I'm into self-healing now."

"What else is there to give up? I've quit smoking and drinking. I don't do drugs. Safe sex only. I could die of boredom."

"They've got us by the balls. That stuff costs a grand a month!"

"I just can't stand to read obituaries anymore."

"You know, stress is the real killer."

"I have something to tell you, love. I'm positive."

"It's only ARC."

"Now the waiting begins."

"Rest in peace, my beloved."

"No rest for the wicked."

"Heard any good AIDS jokes lately?"

"Until there's a cure, there's education."

"You wouldn't dare teach that filth to my children!"

"Abstinence is the only sure bet."

"I'm okay, so far."

"Invisible—again."

"AIDS? Yesterday's news."

"We can't stay depressed forever."

"All my friends are dead."

"Sure they educate—after ten P.M. on PBS."

"This sort of thing brings out every weirdo with an ax to grind."

"And just what do you think we've learned?"

"You sure find out who your friends are—were."

"I'll be here until I die. Can't work. Money's gone."

"Fourth trip to emergency. This is probably the last."

"You know, they buried him away from everybody else. It was that or cremation."

"White gays are getting all the help."

"Yes, they forgave him just before he died. Can you fathom it? *They forgave him.*"

"Every zit, every sniffle, I panic."

"Once can't hurt."

"She went to jail for passing out needles?"

"Thou shalt not is more important than Thou shalt not *whatever.*"

"One step closer to a cure, says the *New England Journal of Medicine.*"

"We can learn so much from this. Better than a war."

"Too expensive to develop."

"Unavailable until thoroughly tested."

"The side effects are worse than the disease."

"Hell, they can't even cure the common cold. And it's a virus, too."

"This thing will bankrupt everyone."

"It's simply a matter of priorities."

"They'll find a way to wriggle out of paying. They always do."

"Never trust the media, one way or another."

"They're stepping all over themselves trying not to offend."

"Sure, I've been tested. What does that prove?"

"They're still trying."

"Maybe not in our lifetime . . . "

"Purely intellectual curiosity."

"I was celibate until I thought I'd go crazy."

"Five years since diagnosis and still going strong. Why?"

"Thanks, Shanti, and all those like you. Unfortunately, thanks is all I can offer."

"Every day's a gift now."

"He finally looks at peace."

"Peace, hell! He's dead! He should be screaming for revenge. We should all be screaming until somebody listens."

"Time softens everything, even resolve."

"All are punished. All are punished!"

Epidemic

Bead, it starts in night,
seed in black earth.
First growing in cells, then
organs, spreading, floating
on blood, in the violet
sea, anemone, medusa.
Soon it owns the body and moves
to the mouth, the holes of secret
access, blows from lip
to lip, dandelion
fluff, invading lover
to lover, mother
to child, the old, even
the dying, no one immune, escaping.
Heart to sinew, skin to bone,
we change in our beds
to things sharp
of vision, long of breath.
There is no cure.

Chapter 11
Bloodstream

As Peter's fever rose he dreamed. A verse came back to him from his teenage years: "He remembered the death of his grandmother. In childhood's spectrum of violence, she remained pure."

He dreamed about the village where his grandmother was raised. They were living in one of the great old Victorian farmhouses with trees and valleys spread out before them—a gray road, like a ribbon, going off into the distance. It was winter in Oregon farm country.

Peter's entire family was now present at the dining table, his grandma at the head. As they celebrated her return from the hospital, all at once her head fell off. Black liquid came oozing out.

"You'll never be the same once you quit drugs and alcohol. You'll be boring and you won't be any fun. You might even die more quickly by giving them up. People have heart attacks when they stop drinking. AIDS sets in after people mend their ways."

Peter squeezed through the opening in the gate. Suddenly he was closed in by trees and a low flint wall. Here a creek ran down through timber and watercress. It was very quiet and still with only the sounds of an owl and the water. A barely perceptible carriage track was cut into the grass. He followed it through the tangled undergrowth. His grandmother's white house loomed up through the trees. He could see the flock of sheep that lived in the house at night, grazing in the thicket by the farm's outbuildings.

"You are only recuperating so that you can go back and get completely bombed for the rest of your life, however long that may be."

Coming into the grape arbor, he went through the little gate, past the sheds. He went into the springhouse that straddled the creek and washed his face there in the chilly water of the rock pool. Crossing the old flower garden, kept irrigated all these years by the creek, he came to the back porch of his grandma's house. Instead of entering, he went around toward the cider mill and past the smokeshed.

"Why were you so hell-bent on destroying yourself, when the very thought of dying of AIDS terrified you?"

Standing in the pasture, near the large stand of pampas grass, with the enormous shadows passing over, Peter looked fixedly at the house. The doors on the porch were gone and the windows broken, but sweet peas and scarlet runner still grew on the pillars. After making his way through the sagging ivy trellis, he went inside. In the musty hallway he ran his fingers along the texture of the wallpaper.

"Watch Peter. Watch him burn. The ball is rolling. How long will the show last? It was already too late. It was too late a long time ago. Laugh, Peter, there's only one choice."

As he came up the familiar lane, the fields below looked like a yellow sea. When he passed the knoll where the church stood blazing white in the shade, a wind was rustling the branches of an oak tree. He looked up at the sky.

"You have had an alcohol and drug problem."

He came bicycling up the narrow dusty road that led through the countryside. The wide dale of green lawns bottomed out below him, and the knoll rose up more and more clearly in the sun. He could see a ridge of pale blue trees. To the left were the purple hills of Grass Valley, Shaniko, and Bakeover. As he turned the bend, the little church ahead glowed white against them.

Peter fell from his bicycle.

Brittle golden leaves blew about him and his bare legs felt damp against the cold grass. He ran his fingers lightly across the hairs of his leg; they looked like golden grass in a field. There was a patch of sun coming through the roof of trees onto the floor of the hillside. He rolled over so that the brightness was not in his eyes.

"You got over your fear of needles quickly, Peter. What are you going to do now? Fill your veins again and be content? Fill up with the Atlantic Ocean? BAM. Suddenly everything feels so different. It's time to float, Peter. Tomorrow never comes. People can smell the drugs coming out of your pores.

"Someone is just going to have to tell your grandmother."

It was raining and he was shaking. He turned over and lay down, his hands folded under his chest. A vein of lightning flashed brightly. It was dusk now, the sky orange. He hoped the raccoons would come out, their eyes shining yellow like a cat's. A great roar of wind was coming up through the tall fir trees. The rain was falling hard and steady on the leaky roof. He clambered down the mossy stairs and took off on his bicycle into the cool rain. For a long distance, he could see the spire of Zena church sticking up crooked in the gray sky.

"Dead people can see you, Peter. Your grandmother is watching you. She always was, and you've been aware of it, too. This enabled you to be proud at moments, and understandably ashamed at others. When a relative died you thought that person would take messages to heaven. But sometimes your grandmother could see for herself. She could see the things you never told anyone."

On the sixth day Peter's fever seemed to decrease. He was able to recognize voices and he could feel the icy cold of a doctor's stethoscope on the cleft of his chest, a blood pressure pad squeezing his arm.

"I dreamed that God was talking to me and that I visited Zena, the place where grandma was born," he said to whomever was in the room.

But then he drifted off again.

"Your mother is in your room, going through it, looking for details. She is looking for clues to find out who you really are."

The voices came back, but Peter's visions had lessened in potency. He was no longer in the country. The landscapes were different now, the topography a conglomeration of all the cityscapes he'd ever known. It was a city of his own creation.

"Do you want to become an alcoholic, like your father?" Then don't go back to New York. Why do you think you got so sick in the first place?"

There were two apple trees and one day they would be large. Peter and his grandmother had planted them on her lot near the golf course. When they came to water them each evening after dinner, Peter would cut down some of the Canadian thistle to make way for a garden. There was one particularly large thistle that grew against the lamppost on the corner. With a sharp object he measured the stock every few weeks and wrote the date on the post. Even then he felt the need to preserve; he sensed that life could change irrevocably.

When his grandmother was dead he came back that September to pick the tomatoes. There weren't very many; he wasn't surprised. He'd learned to accept disappointment. Perhaps neighbors had stolen them.

Although his mother had sold the lot several years ago and a house had been built over their garden, Peter still, in his imagination, could see their lot as it was. He could also imagine the house that his grandmother would have built for them. It would have been in the Roman style with the windows facing an inner courtyard.

"Grandma, can I have a loft in my bedroom?"
"You sure can. We can make it however you want."

Peter's throat was parched. It was so dry that when he swallowed it tickled and he coughed.

When he opened his eyes he couldn't remember where he was. He could see Sara dancing animatedly on a lawn, ducking the water from the sprinkler system that piped water from the lake to the backyard. She was ten years old, the age when he loved her most. Sara was a sweet girl. He loved her. Peter awoke, tears streaming down his face. He pulled the blankets up over his head and dreamed about a particular spot in the trees behind his parents' old house where he had grown up. Immediately after his grandmother died, he'd sat there on the pine-needle floor and didn't know what to do with himself. He brought his sister there once, and they buried a bird in a silver music box they improvised as a coffin.

From that spot in the trees he could see the road, the house, the lawns, and the bamboo garden. Memories came to him quickly, flashing like lightning. Shame. Humiliation. Anger. Love. Is this what is meant by life that passes before one's eyes upon death?

His visions became more and more chaotic. Even with great effort he could not conjure up his grandmother's birthplace, the narrow backroads, the old schoolhouse, the spring where gypsies had camped and where babies were stolen. All he could see was rain. It was raining on the lake.

"Just look, it's raining pitchforks and black babies"—now the voice of his great-grandmother from Kansas.

He awoke. He was icy cold.

When his friend wasn't looking Peter threw a stone at the church's window. It shattered. "Why didn't you tell me you were going to do that? I would have thrown one, too."

From their lookout point in the trees Peter and his school friend could see the cars from the grade school. They collected the rotting apples from the orchard and made a stack of them. When a car passed Peter and his friend would throw an apple. Peter always threw the hardest.

"My son can no longer spend the afternoons with Peter. It's not that Peter is a bad boy, it's just that together they bring out the rebel in each other." It wasn't the first time a mother had said it.

"Pyromania: The uncontrollable impulse to start fires."
Peter liked to watch things burn as a kid—dolls disfigured, toy cars melted.

"Your grandmother died because you were bad."
"But I'm not bad. I'm just sensitive. My puberty was more violent. I was trying to deal with the pressures my father's alcoholism was having on me."
"An excuse."

In the forest across the street from where Peter grew up there was a log. On that log Peter and a friend had smoked their first cigarettes and gotten dizzy and sick. Drugs came years later. In that forest he had seen a neighbor boy running naked. Things happened in these woods. Teenagers drank beer, girls got pregnant.

"A drug addict, alcoholic, deceitful sexual pervert, dying of a disease of the morals. Who would have thought it then, yet clearly the path had been marked." The voice in Peter's head was speaking again.
"Oh, shut up," he told it.

"You broke your mother's heart."
"Stop it."

The fever continued to pulsate through him. He no longer tried to fight it or the thoughts that passed through his mind. The dark lids of his eyes were movie screens. He let go . . .

"What about the sterling your mother claimed you stole from her and sold to satisfy a drug urge, to go to bars and meet your kind of people?"
"The silver belonged to someone my mother hated."
"She felt you betrayed her. You were showing her your utter contempt for the sanctity of family life."
"What good is all this? It isn't true."
"That afternoon when you daydreamed that your grandmother died in a car accident? Do you remember? Your evil thoughts are what made her die a month later."
"But I thought it was God preparing me for her death."
"It wasn't."

In the darkness Peter, as a child, believed he could see faces in the patterns of the tree branches. From his window the trees stood out, long tree trunks that shot up into the sky, taller than skyscrapers. Some day, he thought, one of them would fall.

In the attic of the house where he was born there was an altar with a brass face.

"You were too young to remember the house in Laurelhurst."
"Then what was I remembering?"

From the big windows that faced the forest, people could easily see inside. "There's a man out there," one night Peter shouted.

"Peter sees things that don't exist."

The fever shifted about like ice glaciers moving inside him. Gradually he came out of it. He was more and more aware of the room he lay in. He was able to confirm that it was daylight, that the sun had come out, that it was his mother who was speaking to him.

Despair

From *Spontaneous Combustion*

My anxiety level was high and it was time to do something about it. I had reached a particular level of anxiety that corresponded to the resonant frequency of my brain: one more day in this state and it would explode. I needed to either elevate it to a frequency that only dogs hear, or decrease it to a reasonable level, so I could focus my anxiety on things like nuclear war, famine, torture in third-world countries, Beirut, Afghanistan, Lebanon, the West Bank, crack, the homeless, and my relationship with my mother. In short, it was time to take the Test.

I decided to take the Test after I discovered by reading articles in the *New York Times* that two former sexual partners of mine had AIDS. The first article dealt with AIDS in the workplace. "Why look! There's Ralph," I said to myself, coughing up breakfast and several unrelated meals from the past two weeks. The second was a human interest story about AZT in action. "Gee, didn't know Mark was on AZT these days," I commented from a supine position on the floor, having just fainted.

I decided to take the Test after reading an article in the *New York Times* in which the New York City health commissioner said that all those with the virus were doomed. The prevailing figures I had been reading stated that approximately 15 percent of those exposed to the virus come down with AIDS within five years of infection. I figured I could wait it out: if I stayed well for five years, I'd be home free. I neglected to consider that at the time the epidemic had only been tracked for five years, and the estimates stopped at five years simply because there were no further data. And now it turned out that by seven years' incubation of the virus, the incidence rose sharply.

I decided to take the Test after reading seventeen well-meaning liberal heterosexual columns in seventeen well-meaning liberal het-

erosexual periodicals in which seventeen well-meaning liberal heterosexual people described how they each underwent their own personal
well-meaning liberal heterosexual hell by taking the Test: their fear
and trepidation, their casual doubts and anxieties, along with their
awkward self-reassurances that it would be extremely unlikely to get a
positive antibody result, although they may have had more than
three sexual experiences with more than two partners in the past
seventeen years and it's conceivable that one of the partners was a
hemophiliac bisexual who did intravenous drugs in between weekly
blood transfusions, and it's conceivable that they were inoculated
with a tetanus vaccine using a needle that had just been used on a
hemophiliac bisexual who did intravenous drugs in between weekly
blood transfusions when they were twelve and stepped on a rusty nail
at Camp Mohonka in the Catskills, and it's conceivable that their
mother could actually be Haitian and there could have been a mixup
at the hospital or the midwife's, and it's conceivable that the blood
transfusion from the heart-lung-kidney-and-thyroid transplant by
Doctor Christiaan Barnard had contained some tainted blood from a
hemophiliac bisexual who did intravenous drugs in between weekly
blood donations. I mean, I appreciated reading the first article where
a well-meaning liberal heterosexual columnist described the trials
and tribulations of taking the Test; and even five articles of well-
meaning liberal heterosexual columnists would have been within the
bounds of propriety and taste; but SEVENTEEN of those abominable
articles just made me want to scream. I had it up to here with these
well-meaning liberal heterosexual assholes so far removed from the
crisis that they could be living on Jupiter. You see, these well-meaning
liberal heterosexual columns all ended the exactly the same way, with
the results sheepishly revealed in the final sentence, almost casually,
nonchalantly: Oh, by the way, I was negative. What was this, I
thought, some fucking dating service?

I decided to take the Test even though I had not had the mean
amount of one thousand five hundred twenty-three sexual partners
in the past ten years that the papers reported from the initial group of
AIDS patients (I was rather shy for my age); even though I had not
undergone what was coyly referred to in the press as traumatic sex
(although in some sense all sex is traumatic) in certain downtown
clubs in the presence of a large audience; even though I had never
been considered what was coyly referred to in the company of my
friends as a "slut" (which is undeniably a relative term).

I decided to take the Test even though it wasn't necessarily the
politically correct thing to do, and certain radical gay columnists in

certain radical gay periodicals were predicting the most unbelievable repercussions: mandatory testing for the HIV antibody; discrimination in insurance, housing, and employment of those who tested positive; closing the borders to aliens who tested positive and at the same time other countries closing the borders to Americans who tested positive; internment camps for those who tested positive. As time passed, a significant portion of these alarmist predictions became realities.

I decided to take the Test even though the local gay paper insisted, virulently, that HTLV-III was *not* the cause (although the virus had been renamed HIV two years earlier by an international committee in an effort to solve a dispute about who had discovered the virus first, an American scientist who discovered the virus in 1984 or a French scientist who discovered the virus in 1983) and the local gay paper was backing the African Swine Fever Virus theory, or the Tertiary Syphilis theory, or the Chronic Epstein-Barr Virus theory, or the Cytomegalovirus theory, or the Track Lighting and Industrial Gray Carpeting and Quiche theory, or the Immune System Overload theory, or the Amyl and Butyl Nitrate theory, or a variation of the Legionnaire's Disease theory in which some contaminant got into the air-conditioning system of the Saint discotheque, or perhaps a new noise virus at a certain frequency had gotten into the sound system, or the Government Germ Warfare theory, where some experiment had leaked, not to be confused with the Government Genocide Theory, where the government deliberately distributed contaminated K-Y lubricant at homosexual gatherings and contaminated needles at shooting galleries, or the Airborne Mosquito theory, or the Toilet Seat theory, or the No Gag Response theory, where male homosexuals as a consequence swallow vast quantities of as-yet unidentified toxins. The local gay paper offered a new and improved conspiracy theory each and every month, and I suppose it was *just my problem* that I couldn't keep up with all of these new trends and fashions in disease consciousness; I mean, I guess I was being pigheaded and stupid to accept a parsimonious explanation that had been offered by our admittedly mendacious government, and maybe I was just too irritable and lazy not to make a concerted effort to keep track of each new crackpot theory (based on a somewhat justifiable paranoia) which more or less ignored all scientific research to date and was generally so incredibly stupid that were the theory to be rated on the Stanford-Binet test of general intelligence I doubt it would be able to tie its own shoelaces unassisted or balance a checkbook or cross the street without being run over by a Mack truck.

I decided to take the Test because I was from a rational background and I decided that it wouldn't kill me to know, even though a friend who had AIDS told me that if I found out I was positive this would create additional stress which would in turn weaken my immune system, thus allowing the virus to replicate, a sort of Heisenberg effect where the knowledge of a situation affects that situation, so in fact, it *could* kill me, a little faster than otherwise, and what would the benefits be of finding out if I were positive because there wasn't a cure and why would it help to know my status if it wouldn't change my behavior because I would continue having safe sex and getting enough rest and eating right and exercising and taking Geritol, I mean vitamins, either way? I told him that if I turned out positive I would brood and contemplate suicide and lose perspective and quit my job and go to Italy and finally learn how to deal with my mother and stop transferring money to my Individual Retirement Account and move it into an insurance policy and only renew magazines by the year and would insist on being paid in a lump sum if I won a lottery as opposed to a twenty-year payment scheme because I would probably be dead in twenty years and the tax benefits would be outweighed by the worldwide cruise through whatever countries still allow HIV-positives to travel and maybe I would take one of those fancy new placebos that everyone is talking about, like active lipids or naltrexone or dextran sulfate or wheat grass juice, or maybe I would see a nutritionist and stop eating sugar and become macrobiotic and then die a lot faster from not eating enough protein, or maybe I would start meditating, or maybe I would finally achieve a sense of spirituality and meaning in my life as it neared the end and drop this worn cloak of cynicism for crystals or Gurdjieff or reincarnation or God or free parking, or maybe I would start writing faster like Anthony Burgess who when misdiagnosed with a brain tumor wrote four novels in a year, or maybe I would have some cosmic revelation earlier because I was ready for it, or maybe I would join a bowling league, or maybe I would just give up. I mean, I operated under the basic premise that ignorance is *not* bliss and why should I stick my head in the sand when I should perfectly well be able to stick the gun in my mouth instead? And then, of course, there was the extremely slim chance that I was, in fact, HIV-negative. Maybe, who knows? I could actually relax for a few minutes. I mean, Rome wasn't built in a day. I'm sure it's nothing that fifteen years of intense psychotherapy couldn't get to the bottom of.

I decided to take the Test because, although I generally don't believe in predestination as opposed to free will, from a logical standpoint we are all born with certain finite constraints: None of us is immortal; hence, none of us has an unlimited number of heartbeats left. Women are born with a finite number of ova, ready to plop down the fallopian tubes at the rate of one every four weeks, from puberty to menopause; similarly, we are each born with a finite number of orgasms to experience, cigarettes to smoke, and lovers to betray. Knowing whether I tested positive or negative could help me determine more precisely what these numbers were. I was just moderately curious to find out what would be a reasonable number of cocktails, nightmares, Lean Cuisines, boyfriends, vacations, apartments, breaths, jobs, and bowel movements to expect in this lifetime. Perhaps if I knew I had only a few sexual relations left, I would avoid intercourse in order to stretch things out?

I decided to take the Test because I had reached the point where I believed that it was a fundamentally irrational act *not* to take the HIV antibody test and after all I *did* graduate from the Massachusetts Institute of Technocracy several eons ago and consequently I still felt a responsibility to behave rationally.

So, nervous like when I was seventeen and in college and still a virgin and went to a drugstore and spent hours studying depilatories and decongestants and diuretics before finally, in a cracked voice, asking the kindly pharmacist for condoms, I picked up the phone and dialed the city AIDS hotline and made an appointment to take the Test at the earliest available time slot, six weeks later. Like a secret agent, I was identified by a numeric code only.

During the next six weeks I did the usual things: made a will, sold my co-op, changed my job, upped my insurance, reconciled with my family, wrote a novel, worked out at the gym seven times a day, had sixteen failed romances, tried to volunteer as an astronaut at NASA so I could experience the relativistic effects of traveling at high speeds (time contracts when approaching the speed of light, thus the six weeks' wait would seem less interminable).

The six weeks wait was an eternity.

That morning ("There's still time to chicken out," said my friend William), I woke up early and took the bus. I had scheduled my appointment for 8:30, when the clinic opened, so I could take the Test, vomit, and then casually waltz into work fashionably late, as usual.

There was no time for breakfast; I didn't want to be late. I took the bus down Ninth Avenue. I had to stand until Forty-second Street. I couldn't concentrate on the *Times*. The bus let me off right in front of the Chelsea Clinic. I hadn't been there since 1980, when I went to get treated for a venereal disease.

Outside several homeless people were sleeping on benches. A man swept debris from the concrete with a broom. The clinic was next to an elementary school, with a jungle gym outside. It was 8:15. The building was closed.

I circled the block. Several sexually responsive individuals had thoughtfully left their used condoms on the sidewalk. It reminded me of the first time I ever set foot in a gay bar, back when I was nineteen in Pasadena, California. I had circled the street seventy-two times before gathering enough courage to enter. I was shy; I wasn't ready to make a lifestyle commitment at that point in time, and I thought entering a gay bar would be an irrevocable step. I mean, they'd all think I was a homosexual.

I had a quick bite to eat at an awful deli on Tenth, surrounded by the harsh accents of the outer boroughs: the snide voices, the know-it-alls, the jokers. How could they joke at a time like this? I wondered. I returned to the clinic, ten minutes late for my 8:30 appointment. Two people were already in front of me. I was given an interesting and informative booklet to read. Why did the print fade the harder I tried to concentrate? The woman at the desk asked for my number and then asked me to make up a new one, tossing the first away. I signed a release form by copying a statement instead of signing: with no signature, no identifying marks were left. Then I had a brief counseling session with a therapist, a woman with dark hair cut butch, a warm and sympathetic lesbian.

"How do you think you were exposed?" she asked.

"I may have forgot to use a condom five or six thousand times back in 1982, before there were rules and regulations to follow."

"Why are you taking the test? What will this knowledge do for you?"

"I thought . . . " I thought this was a test, and the right answer would be judicious and thoughtful and beneficial to humanity, " . . . that I might be able to help further the cause of science and medical research by becoming an experimental subject, should I test positive."

"I wouldn't if I were you," she counseled. "They have double-blind experiments. For all you know you could be eating sugar pills. And what's worse, you may be on some toxic drug. Suppose you're in a study and they find out another more promising drug. You can't switch." Then she told me about macrobiotic diets and stress reduction and homemade AL721.

"That's a bit drastic for me. I mean, should I give up meat just to live another six months?" There was this trade-off between sex and life, between red meat and a few more years. Why should I have to be making these choices?

"For the next two weeks, I want you to act as if you have already tested positive," she advised. "Prepare yourself." Did she know something that I didn't know? Why couldn't I enjoy my last few possibly blissful weeks and be relatively stress-free (although by this time my anxiety meter reading was off the scale)? I made an appointment for two weeks later to get my results.

The Indian medical assistant looked up from his textbook and put on two pairs of red plastic gloves. "Give me your arm," he instructed. Carefully, he stuck me with the needle and filled a test tube with my blood, then wrapped the gloves around the sample for safety. I wondered how he could do this all day. How could he stand it?

That night I found out that Gordon had died in the afternoon. My first reaction was, "See what you get for taking the test?" Although I eventually convinced myself there was no cause-and-effect relationship between the two events, still, I felt it was not a good sign.

"You can always just take it and not bother getting the results," said my friend William. "You can back out at any time."

The next day I called Richard in California.

"If it turns out I'm positive, I'm going to take the next plane out of here and get a cab to your apartment and knock on your door and you'll answer and I'll say, 'Thanks,' and pull out my pearl-handled revolver from my purse and shoot you dead."

"Come on, Benjamin, I didn't necessarily infect you; it could be anyone of thousands."

"I know it would be you. Who else fucked me with such relish and regularity? Who else do I know with lymphadenopathy from 1982? Besides, it's easier for me to deal with when I can pinpoint the blame on someone else."

"You should be here in San Francisco. We're so specialized here we even have groups for people who are waiting to find out whether they tested positive or negative."

"Two week groups?"

"That's right."

"If only they came out with the safe sex regulations two months earlier, I'd still be alive."

"You *are* alive, Benjamin."

"You know what I mean." Was it better to have loved and gotten infected than never to have loved at all? Was I even capable of love? Who knows?

Instead of San Francisco, I went to Provincetown, the only gay mecca to which I hadn't yet made a pilgrimage (I had already been to Key West and West Hollywood). I had another disastrous safe-sex romance, and then I got too much sun and not enough sleep, because there was sand in my weekend lover's bed, and being the Jewish American Princess that I am, it felt just like a pea; I mean, the pullout mattress hadn't been turned since the War between the States, so I tossed and turned and created my own forcefield of anxiety, and so my face decided to punish me with a minor outbreak of herpes which, in turn, got infected with impetigo which, in turn, increased my level of anxiety so the herpes got worse and worse and by the time it had reached its nadir I looked more or less like Jeff Goldblum in the remake of *The Fly,* and this was not during the first half hour of this picture, this was *serious* skin disorder. So I went to my doctor, who had fled the city that January because of burn-out from the AIDS crisis, and saw his cruel replacement, a cold and inefficient reptile who misdiagnosed me with shingles, a disease that typically affects only half the face, whereas my face was a *complete* disaster area. And then this lizard had the tact to tell me that I should definitely take the HIV antibody test because shingles was one of those opportunistic infections that tends to strike people with lowered immunities and he said that he felt there was a 90 percent chance that I would be positive. At which point I told my own personal nominee for Mister Compassion and Tact of 1987 that I had already taken the test and as a matter of fact was expecting my results the following day.

I went back to the Chelsea Clinic for my results, looking like the Creature from the Black Lagoon. Guess what? Unlike the seventeen well-meaning liberal heterosexual columnists in the seventeen well-meaning liberal heterosexual periodicals, I turned out to be positive. Hold the presses! This had to be front-page news. I was going to make the *Guiness Book of World Records,* the cover of *Time, Esquire,* and *Woman's Wear Daily,* as the first columnist to turn out positive in the history of civilization, and parlay this into immediate financial gain, a guest spot on "Hollywood Squares," a bit part in "Miami Vice," when I realized I would be dead before the residuals came because my life expectancy wasn't quite so long as it was even a week ago. You know, here I was, thinking like an actuary. I decided it was time to get a television set, something I had been struggling successfully against acquiring for the past ten years, along with a VCR so that when my apartment was converted into a sanatorium I'd be able to amuse myself. I didn't go whole-hog, however: cable would have to wait.

And oddly enough I fell into this deep funk.

I had a friend who was nice and supportive, and after I took the Test and got the results he got really mad at me because I was depressed because what did I expect? And didn't I realize the likelihood of being positive? And what difference did it make anyway? And I told him it was the doom, the absolute doom that got to me, and he said didn't you know about that before, you imbecile? And I said this is the sort of thing you can't really figure out what your reaction will be until you do it, and I tried to explain to him about the Heisenberg principle but he had math anxiety in a bad way so he stuffed his fingers into his ears and said I don't want to listen. And of course a couple of months later he took the Test anyway, on the advice of his doctor who told him that if he had high blood pressure wouldn't he want to know if he was at risk of a heart attack, even if it was only a 10 percent chance? And he was negative. And another friend who had moved to Japan three years ago to evade the AIDS crisis and the Reagan administration and also because something snapped in his brain when he turned thirty and he—with no prior warning—became a wizened and depraved rice queen who had traveled nine thousand miles just to get laid; well, he took the Test and he was negative too. And then another friend who had, according to conservative estimates, sucked every Negro penis in the tri-state area between the ages of sixteen and forty-five in subways, tearooms, trucks, changing rooms, and the back seats of cars; well, he took the Test, and he was negative too. And part of me, since misery loves company, wanted just one close friend to be positive too, but the sensible part of me, you know, the part that still has occasional communication with my cerebral cortex, said, "Thank God they're negative," using the expletive for effect since, thank God, my experience had not changed me so profoundly that I was no longer an atheist.

So this is what I do: I go on with my life. I go to ACT UP meetings, never saying a word, and end up more stressed-out than I was before; I go to demonstrations and scream myself hoarse and then visit my new primary health care practitioner who, unlike the lizard, gives me hugs and prescribes medication for my sore throat and my various and sundry female disorders; I get my T-cell count taken every three months; I go to a few Body Positive meetings for HIV-positives and attend a group rap session that is headed by a psychopath and shortly thereafter drop out because once again my stress-level has tripled during the course of the meeting; and I want to end the AIDS crisis and stop the government logjam of red tape and paperwork and there should be some sort of cure in the near future and the only thing is will I still be alive; and I'm wary of the macrobiotic diets and crystals and lipids and other untested and unverified treatments but at the same time I'm afraid to do absolutely nothing, maybe I'm paralyzed by inertia and fear, I don't know, and I don't want to take AZT when the T-cell count drops below 200 because it's highly toxic but at the same time I know it can't be all bad because some more insane people at the local gay paper want to charge all doctors with malpractice for prescribing it. And I take acyclivoir for my herpes twice daily to prevent recurrences because herpes is particularly bad for the immune system and I'm avoiding the sun: this summer I'm going to be a porcelain goddess, a pale creature of the night. And sex: what about sex? When I see a guy I've been flirting with for the past four years, what do I say? What are the rules? Should this be broadcast? Are there any tactful ways of telling the relatives? How can I have sex with someone without telling? Does it matter if the sex is absolutely safe? What do I say when I meet someone new: would you like to have sex with someone who may or may not have a fatal disease?

And now I never sleep through the night; I always wake up at three or four, tense, filled with anxiety. Like Dorothy in the *Wizard of Oz,* I sit, watching helplessly as my T-cell count drops every three months, the sands of time running out.

Once I awoke from a wet dream, swimming in a sea of infected sperm; I leapt out of the bed to wipe it all up, quickly (how does one stem the tide, the flow?). And one day I was sitting at a coffee shop and my nose began to bleed spontaneously. I hadn't had a nosebleed in years. The blood dripped bright red onto the plate, onto the napkin. All I could think of was infection and disease. All I could think of was the virus that was coursing through my blood. I blotted it out with the napkin and sat there ashamed, frightened, in despair.

Spring and Fall

"No, no, I'm perfectly all right," said James. "I just get a bit tired at six o'clock, seven o'clock."

"Perhaps I should go," Brendan said. He looked anxious and uncomfortable. He had moved two days before into a house at the other end of the street and had popped in to say hello to these old friends he'd not seen in a while, James and his lover, Owen. He was surprised to find James in bed after hearing of James's recovery—on his feet again and fit as a fiddle, a mutual acquaintance assured him.

"He really is all right," said Owen, who was hovering in the doorway: tall, big-boned, and attractive. Such a contrast to James, a wiry, puckish man; thinner, Brendan decided, than he had been. Weight loss, of course, was always one of the problems.

"We'll have drinks in here," James said. "Swigging alcohol dressed in only a duvet cover is pleasantly *camp.*"

"Makes him feel he's holding court," said Owen, smiling at his lover. He left the room and called out from the kitchen, "Gins and tonics for everyone, OK?"

"It's hot," Brendan said. "Hot, hot, hot!" It was indeed: the sultriest day of the sultriest of summers. He was wearing shorts and a T-shirt—as was Owen; their appraisal of each other's naked legs had been, so James should not be upset, very surreptitious, but Brendan was aware of the direction of Owen's glance. James was aware of it too, though they didn't realize that.

"Sit on the bed, Brendan. I had to put up with a bout of PCP at Easter—"

"So I heard."

"—and it's made me a bit deaf in one ear. And given me tinnitus. If you're not right beside me I won't understand what you're saying." He laughed. "Still ... even that has compensations! I have a disability sticker on my car now, so I can park on all the yellow lines and not get wheel-clamped. And I have a half-fare travel pass for the trains and buses—as if I was an old-age pensioner. I'm only twenty-nine!"

"Same age as me."

"And Owen. He's not even positive! And here I am, a fully fledged PWA. Incredible . . . His cock must be made of galvanized iron."

Owen returned with the gins. "This is strong!" Brendan exclaimed. "Just as well I don't have to drive home!"

"How's the new flat?" Owen asked. "Everything sorted out?"

"Cardboard cartons all over the place; I can hardly move in the sitting room. I've unpacked my clothes and fixed up the kitchen, but that's as far as I've got." He paused and stared out of the window. "Islington: I shall like it here."

"This is a good street. Regency; elegant and expensive. With quite a few other gay couples, also rich in pink pounds."

"Irredeemably middle class," James said.

"Ignore him, Brendan. James is always teasing me about my being middle class. Because I wear a suit and a tie when I go to work. Who doesn't in the City?"

"It's the rolled umbrella that gets me."

"Nonsense."

"And voting Tory."

"I voted Democrat—"

"Worse than Tory. Particularly as our M.P., that nice Mr. Smith, is the one and only out gay M.P. in the whole of Britain."

"But he's a socialist."

"So what?"

Owen didn't reply. It was a well-rehearsed routine, this: they had been over it many times, and it signified nothing. In fact, James found Owen's middle class–ness rather endearing: it was a kind of naïveté, a relic of childhood and home, and had little to do with umbrellas and supporting the Democrats. Owen was still very much in tune with his background—a leafy, well-off suburb of southwest London and parents who accepted their only child's sexual orientation with surprising ease and graciousness. Owen's discovery in adolescence that he was gay had never led him to question the established order of things, or to learn much from the experiences of other people: from the age of nineteen until he was twenty-four—when he met James—he'd screwed with dozens of men (suburban southwest London would not have approved of *that*), but they left little impression on him. With James he'd made a commitment, "settled down." It was a marriage, and gay marriage to Owen was the exact equivalent of its heterosexual counterpart.

Fidelity also suited James, who had no more desire than Owen to sleep around: he too, at twenty-four, had done his fair share—but in one of those torrid, sweaty sessions before Owen came into his life he'd contracted the virus. He did not think, however, that a relationship between two men was at all like a straight marriage, and he had long since rejected everything to do with the values, assumptions, and demands of his own background, which was remarkably similar to Owen's. James saw his lover's clinging to the certainties of the past as an attractive innocence. And he felt that, despite his hunky exterior, Owen would always need care and protection.

"Don't you like Islington?" Brendan asked.

"Well . . . it's somewhere to live, I suppose," James replied.

Owen tut-tutted. "He adores it! He couldn't imagine living anywhere else! The boutiques and bistros, the delicatessens, and every wine shop you go into there are queens with poodles buying Chateau Mouton Rothschild . . . Joe Orton's house two streets down, blue plaque and so on."

James stuck out his tongue at Owen, then smiled. "I admit it . . . I'd hate to live elsewhere."

"The only problem is we're a long way from the hospital."

"Which one do you go to?" Brendan asked.

"St. Mary's," James said.

"I forgot the ice." Owen stood up.

"Is there a lover unpacking the cardboard cartons while you're out?" James wanted to know. "Or slaving over a superb candle-lit dinner for two?"

"The longest relationship I've ever had," Brendan said, "lasted three months; the second and third months were a battleground. I used to think there was something peculiar about me—we're so indoctrinated into thinking the status of being single is inferior to being part of a couple. Once upon a time I envied you two! Not now. I enjoy being single . . . I couldn't cope with a lover. A live-in man . . . No!"

"Owen couldn't cope without. He'll fall to bits when I'm dead."

"That's . . . that's years off."

"You shouldn't talk that way!" James said, sharply. "You're just covering your own backside."

Brendan, struck by the truth of this, said, "I'm sorry."

"Still . . . I imagine you get your men."

"You have to be so careful these days. Which . . . sometimes spoils the thrill of it. But . . . I don't go short."

James nodded. "Man as good looking as you."

Owen, coming back into the room with the ice, said to himself, yes, indeed Brendan *was* cute; curly blond and impish, skin dark from the summer's heat. How long had they known one another? Seven years, eight? In the time before James they had gone out on the scene together, sisters. If they each found a man for the night, they compared notes on the phone the next day. Brendan's men, Owen recalled, were a catalogue of absurd disasters—the stunning Afro hair of a Frenchman that proved to be a wig; a mad, drunk ballet dancer who had offered as a lubricant a tub of polyunsaturated margarine; and the only man who ever whisked Brendan away in a Porsche was arrested by the police for drunk driving before they'd arrived at the promised Docklands penthouse. When Owen first met Brendan he was aware that they found each other attractive, but they had never done anything about it. The question hung in the air unanswered for a few weeks and was then made redundant by the warmth of friendship. Though Brendan also worked in the City, they didn't see a lot of each other these days—a dinner party, perhaps, every six months or so; that was all.

"Do you have a cigarette?" Owen asked. "I've run out."

"You're losing your memory," Brendan answered. "I don't smoke."

"And I gave it up," said James. "After the pneumocystis carinii."

"You're very frank," Brendan said to him. "And cheerful. I'd thought . . . to be honest . . . that I'd find doom and gloom. Or a façade of nothing is wrong."

"You know us better!" James was scornful. "I've been perfectly frank from the start. Three reasons: First, no landlord can chuck me out of this house—we own it jointly, Owen and me. Second, I can't get the sack from work because I don't work anymore. I'm not fit enough. I resigned. So . . . unlike many people . . . I've nothing to lose. And third, I still remember the joy of coming out of the closet ten years ago. No more pretences, no more lies! To hide the fact that I have AIDS would be like creeping into that closet again. I feel sad . . . and a bit contemptuous . . . when I hear about those guys—the rich and famous as well as the quite ordinary—who we're told have died from leukemia or cancer of the stomach when everyone knows it was an AIDS-related disease. It diminishes all of us! Implies we should feel ashamed of what's happened! Plays the dirty tabloid press at their own vicious games. Look what they did to Ian Charleson! *I* won't be part of that. If anyone writes my obituary, which I doubt they will because I've never done anything worth recording, I want it stated in print: 'He died of pneumocystis carinii pneumonia, an opportunistic infection caused by AIDS.' Assuming it is PCP that carries me off."

"Quite a speech," Owen said, smiling. "You'll exhaust yourself."

"Well . . . "

"Do you manage to go out much?" Brendan asked.

"If somebody asks us to dinner I psych myself up and enjoy the occasion as much as I ever did. But we don't get to the theater now, or concerts . . . I can't hear what's going on."

"We struggle down to the gay pub two or three nights a week," Owen said.

"Struggle! Don't listen to him . . . We troll. We swish."

"To the King Ethelred the Unready?" Brendan asked.

"Nice pub. Nice crowd too. But I think the name is a mistake . . . There's at least one *extremely* cute barman in there who's more than ready. Every time we go in he mentally strips Owen naked . . . You can see him doing it. Owen gets so embarrassed."

"I do not! I take it as a compliment!"

"If I tell you you're embarrassed," James said with a grin and a flick of the wrist, "then you *are* embarrassed."

"James is enjoying himself," Owen said, almost serenely.

"If the barman is as cute as you say he is," Brendan said, "and he mentally takes off all *my* clothes . . . then I'll chat him up. I'm ready for a little something or other. Almost overdue."

"Overdue!" James laughed. "The word reminds me of the four forty-five from Plymouth."

"The what?"

"Yes . . . it was in the first days of our relationship . . . We'd only known each other a fortnight, and I went down to Plymouth on business, a whole, agonizing week without Owen! He had to be in London . . . We arranged to meet half-way, on the Friday night, for a dirty weekend in Bath. I caught the four forty-five train, and it was held up for hours! It was so late I was sure he'd have gone; he *loathes* unpunctuality. My little heart was going pit-a-pat and I kept running to the loo . . . I rushed out of Bath station and there he was. 'Thank God you're still here!' he said. 'I've only just arrived; the five o'clock from Paddington broke down at Slough and we had to wait for another engine.'" James leaned back on the pillows and smiled. "Then he said . . . it was the first time . . . 'I love you.'" Owen took his hand and they looked at each other affectionately: old married couple.

"And was it a dirty weekend?"

"Well . . . we went down into the Roman bath . . . visited the cathedral . . . saw the Jane Austen relics, and Landsdowne Crescent, Cavendish Crescent, and Royal Circus . . . ate some good meals . . . But I do seem to remember Owen had quite enough time to explore all my orifices very thoroughly. And very efficiently."

"James!" Owen was shocked. "What a way to put it!"

"Why not?"

"It's . . . private!"

"Middle class!" James teased. "Middle class!"

"Oh . . . get stuffed!"

"I did!"

Brendan finished his drink, then looked at his watch. "I must go," he said. "Dinner to find. And cardboard cartons rather than orifices to explore."

"I'll walk along with you," Owen said. "I need some cigarettes."

Outside, the full blast of the heat rose from the pavement. The little terraces of white houses seemed tired, punished by the tropical weather, but patient: we will endure, their message appeared to be; we'll outlast you. "It's as hot as Egypt," Brendan said. Then, after a pause, "How long does he have?"

"James?" Owen shrugged his shoulders. "He's well enough . . . this week . . . I don't think about it."

"He's a little . . . waspish."

"You would be too. He . . . doesn't enjoy this heat."

"And you . . . How do you cope?"

"I don't think about it," Owen said again. "I get on with whatever is next. How else does one cope? Work . . . keeping the rooms tidy . . . seeing to his needs."

Brendan waited while he went into the tobacconist's. "Would you like to come in and see the flat?"

"Yes. Why not?"

The entire floor of the sitting room, as Brendan had said, was filled with cardboard cartons. And suitcases, books, the stereo, the television, the video, squash rackets, lampshades, pictures, cushions: the accumulations of a life. They stared at it all in silence. I suppose my house will soon look like this, Owen said to himself. Sorting through James's things. "It will be OK when I've got myself organized," Brendan said. "The problem is I can't decide whether I should unpack first, then paint the walls, or do it the other way round."

"Unpack," Owen said. "That's what we did."

Brendan cleared a path through the debris. "This is the view," he said.

They stood at the window and gazed out: their shoulders touched.

Plane trees, leaves already weary; parked cars, colored front doors, black railings. A dog sniffing at litter. An old woman lugging two heavy carrier bags. Dust, dust, dust.

Brendan's right hand was stroking Owen's skin near the bottom of his shorts. Owen was instantly erect, shaking with desire. He had not had sex for weeks—James had neither the urge nor the energy; only wanted to be held. Owen kissed Brendan on the mouth, a long, passionate kiss that seemed exquisitely gentle and complex. But when he realized that his hand was on Brendan's cock, and that Brendan's was on his, he pulled away. "No," he said. "Not now. It would be ... a betrayal." He left hurriedly and ran back home.

"You took your time," James said.

Owen blushed, and aware that guilt was evident in his face, he said, "He asked me in to see the flat. We didn't ... "

James laughed. "No, I don't imagine for one second you did. I know how long you take and that would have been uncharacteristically quick! But ... you have an erection. I can see it." Owen said nothing. "Come here," he went on. "Hold me. Kiss me."

Owen obeyed.

"We have to face it," James said. "There isn't a huge amount of time. So many last things ... The last time we went to a concert ... The last time we made love. You have to begin to think of yourself, Owen. You and Brendan obviously fancy each other ... Sleep with him if you want. I shan't mind ... really I shan't ... It's too late for me to worry about something like that."

Owen's response was to burst into tears, floods of uncontrollable tears, weeks and weeks of emotion held in check now pouring out. So James held him—not his role during the previous twelve months—and kissed him, caressed his hair.

Eventually Owen stopped. "I'm confused," he said. "I'm not sure what I'm crying about."

"Yourself," James answered. "The blight man was born for. It is Margaret you mourn for."

They stared at each other: a long moment, both of them aghast because they knew that Owen, finally, after all the years with James, had lost his innocence.

The Federal Bureau of Blood Inspection

March 2000

Morris sits in the waiting room of the Columbia Hospital for Women, alternately flipping through an aging copy of *Parents* magazine and looking at his watch. His wife, Ellen, and their baby, Celia, are with the doctor. Nervously, he glances down; the staff meeting is at three, and as campaign manager he has to be there. The senator wants a final agenda for the next month of what is becoming a tense and unpredictable presidential race.

"Mr. Apter," the nurse's voice is leaden, "the doctor wants to speak with you."

At the end of a long, gray corridor, Morris is greeted by the pediatrician's outstretched hand. "Hello, Morris, how's the campaign going? Think the Democrats have a chance this time?"

"Absolutely. We're going to win this one." He smiles at Ellen and notices how pale she looks. He steps to her side and puts his arm around her shoulder. "What's the matter, honey?" She doesn't answer.

"Morris, Celia isn't gaining weight. She's not growing. I don't have an explanation yet. We need to run some tests." The doctor doesn't look at him.

"What tests? Is this serious?"

"Probably not. Could be a minor infection." The doctor shifts his eyes to Ellen. "But I want to test for HIV."

"HIV!" Morris almost laughs. "Celia can't have AIDS."

"We have to rule it out. Let's talk after the test is done." The doctor stands up, indicating the appointment is over.

As they walk to the parking garage Morris watches Ellen's red hair brighten in the spring sun, her incredible hair that first attracted him. She turns toward him, the baby in her arms, her eyes flooding with tears. He hugs them, murmuring words of comfort. "Don't cry,

El. He just wants to rule it out. They test for everything these days."

"Mo, I'm scared. Really scared." Tears stream down her cheeks.

"This is merely routine, honey. Celia doesn't have AIDS. It's not possible."

"We have to talk, Morris."

"Tonight, honey. I'm late for the staff meeting."

"What?" She glares at him with a look that makes him feel instantly guilty.

"Come on, El," he pleads. "Celia's going to be fine. You knew when I took this job I'd be working day and night until the election. Be realistic."

"Realistic! Didn't you hear what he said? He said AIDS!" She chokes on the word.

"Okay, okay. Calm down. I'll call George. He can get things started." Fear creeps up his spine. He stares at the cherry blossoms along Rock Creek Parkway. In the rearview mirror he watches Celia sleep.

They turn into the driveway of their new house in McClean. The dog sits in the window, wagging his tail. A chewed-up bedroom slipper lies in the foyer. Morris lets the dog into the backyard while Ellen settles Celia into her crib. The coffee is still warm. Morris reaches for two mugs and pours them each a cup. The porcelain cow his aunt gave them is empty. When he fills it, this normal task heightens his fear and a growing sense of unreality. He picks up the *Washington Post*. The headline, "AIDS Drug Found Too Toxic for Majority of Patients," announces the FDA's revision of guidelines for human vaccine trials. Neither vaccination nor drug treatment has been successful; 700,000 are dying and a million deaths are predicted for 2000. One of his staffers has been in and out of the hospital. His single friends discuss it incessantly, but for him AIDS is only a depressing fact of other peoples' lives. Luckily, he met Ellen when he did. Monogamy without condoms, they used to joke, a practice they could live with.

Ellen strokes the soft wisps of hair on Celia's head and rearranges her blankets. She puts the music-box bunny in the crib and winds it up. It plays "you are my sunshine." She's such a beautiful baby, Ellen thinks, pulling the handmade quilt over Celia's shoulders and patting her tiny back. It is inconceivable that anything bad could happen to her.

Ellen stays beside the crib a long time. Morris comes to the doorway and gestures for her to join him. He puts his arm around her and leads her down the hallway, wishing he could make the last two hours disappear. "George is covering for me for an hour."

"I'm sorry, Mo. I'm okay now. You can go."

"Here, have a cup of coffee. Listen, honey, we both know Celia can't have the AIDS virus. Don't worry about it."

Ellen collapses into the kitchen chair like a rag doll. "She's sick, Mo. Something is making her sick. I can't help worrying. Anyway, the doctor asked me some disturbing questions. Questions about our sex lives, and if either of us used drugs. He seems to think one of us could have the AIDS virus. It's unbelievable."

His sense of disbelief is turning to anger. This can't happen to them. Neither have had blood transfusions, or shot up drugs, or had gay lovers. They talked about past lovers on their third date. "Ellen, what exactly did he say? How far back can this go?" He reaches for the phone.

"Don't call him." She knows what he's feeling.

"Why not?"

"It's your turn to calm down, Mo. Think about Celia. She sleeps more than other babies. She isn't gaining weight. She's had a cold since the day she was born. It's possible, isn't it? Tell me it isn't. Please." She starts to cry again.

"It isn't possible, El." The water faucet drips. He gets up to turn it off. Celia's sea-blue eyes gaze back at him like an apparition in the kitchen window. Nausea swells in his stomach. His muscles stiffen until they ache.

"Have you slept with anyone since we married?" Ellen's voice is flat, devoid of blame or anger.

"I haven't slept with another woman since the first time I slept with you." Placing his chair so that their knees are touching, he looks directly into her eyes. He reaches out and runs his fingers over her tear-stained cheek. "I love you. I love Celia. You know how much I love you both."

She stares at him. "What's going to happen to us, Mo?"

January 2001

It is bitter cold. A dust of snow covers the frozen earth. They stand with their friends beside the small hole in the ground. The gravediggers shift, restless, around their shovels several feet away. Celia's coffin is slowly lowered into the grave. The rabbi says a few words. Ellen tosses the music-box bunny onto the coffin. Morris is rigid with grief. They don't hold hands. Their friends are crying, but they are beyond tears. Ellen steps back and notices three other funerals taking place. "Everyone is dying," she mutters.

Morris and Ellen have agreed to separate. Ellen is staying in the house where they struggled for Celia's life. Morris is moving to a studio apartment on Capitol Hill. They are both seropositive, but neither cares. Celia's death overshadows everything. They have lived for almost a year in a nightmare, and in spite of the best efforts of their friends and therapists nothing anyone says penetrates their pain.

After the funeral Ellen goes into Celia's empty room. She shakes out the blankets and folds them neatly across the bottom of the crib. She puts the unused Pampers back in the box and lines all the stuffed animals in a row across the dresser. Morris stands in the door and observes. He aches to touch her. She is oblivious to comfort but acknowledges his presence. "Why don't you make coffee? The others will be here with the food soon. Put out the good china and silver. I want to have a proper sort of reception. She was only eighteen months old, but . . . " Ellen's eyes fill with tears. She clutches a teddy bear to her chest, then sinks to the floor. "Oh God, oh God, Morris. Oh God. I want my baby back."

He goes to her and holds her. His tears fall into her hair, but no words come.

August 1995

Ellen loves the weight of Washington's hot, humid August days. She sits in her Dupont Circle office, waiting for her next patient and watching the passersby out her window. Her private practice is flourishing. Her Adams Morgan apartment is finally furnished. Her student loans are paid. She is splurging this summer on clothes, a health club, and a Georgetown hairdresser. As an unattached, professional woman she is invited to countless summer parties. She dates several men at once and often overbooks herself, a relic of past insecurity and lonely college years. Then she was thirty pounds overweight, wore ugly glasses, and devoted herself to psychology. Now she has everything she dreamt of, everything she worked for. She muses, My tortured adolescence is finally over. Work hard, play hard.

The phone rings. She pushes her long hair back and answers it. "Dr. Walker speaking."

"Hi. Mark Rogers here. We danced last week at d.c. space, remember?"

"Sure. You're the lawyer."

"Right. I wondered, are you free on Saturday night? There's a dancing party on Reno Road."

"Saturday night . . . ," she hesitates. She has a date with a financial analyst she met at an investment seminar, but she isn't enthusiastic about him. Mark is a handsome, blond lawyer. "I think so, but I'll have to call you back."

"Fine. Can you let me know tonight? I'm looking forward to some more wild dancing." His voice is seductive.

"Yeah," she laughs, "that was fun. What's your phone number?"

She spends the evening on the phone rearranging her weekend, squeezing five dates into two days.

Her first date with Mark is more eventful than she expected. After a romantic dinner they go to the party and dance the night away. Later at his apartment they make love. Sex on the first date is on her list of DON'T EVERS, but it happens. Afterward, Mark tells her the story of his unsuccessful marriage. She feels a twinge of regret and dismay while listening to him. He tells her of several affairs since his divorce. With the AIDS crisis looming, her carelessness leaves her ill at ease. She didn't mention using a condom, which she usually did. Swept away in the heat of passion she didn't think. What are the chances? she's thinking now. Infinitesimally small. But she promises herself she will never do this again.

September 1995

"Hey, Mo, you gonna watch the goddamn game or not?" George yells from the cramped and cluttered living room to Morris, who has taken a phone call in his equally messy bedroom. The usual crowd is gathered to watch the Redskins play Dallas. Morris has been on the phone with Linda for nearly an hour. She always calls at gametime. Everyone urges him to end it with her, but he won't. Even though she lives with another man, Morris continues to see her. He irrationally believes they will end up together.

Bob goes to the well-worn refrigerator, pulls out a six-pack, and passes it around. Finally, Morris mopes out of the bedroom.

"Cheer up, Mo," says Bob. "Christ, we've all got problems. I met the hottest woman last week. We're in bed, and she says to me, 'Got a rubber?' I say, 'No, baby, I'm clean.' She says, 'No rubber, no sex.' She puts on her clothes and shows me the door. A real pisser. What the fuck do women want anyway?"

"Let's see . . . ," Mo rubs his chin. "Money. Power. Good looks. Security. And now, safe sex."

"No such thing as safe sex," George interjects.

"Cut the moaning, asshole. Take a trip to the drug store."

"That's pure high school. Any of you carry rubbers around?"

"Me. I wear two at a time. When I slip one off I get this incredible surge of freedom."

Laughter erupts. "Hey, Mark, that redhead at Margie's party—who is she? She's almost as gorgeous as you. Look at that play! Those idiots can't fight their way out of a wet paper bag. Where the fuck is George Allen when you need him?"

Mark smiles at Bill, the compliment not passing him by. "Ellen Walker, Ph.D. Not bad, huh? A great dancer."

Bill grins. "Yeah. Women have their moments. Nothing better than a good, home-cooked dinner, cuddling in front of the tube, clean socks and underwear, a soft shoulder to cry on, once in a while." He winks at Mark. The others are lost in the game.

"Hey, where's the pizza?"

"I'll go," Mark volunteers.

"I'll keep you company." Bill gets up and collects five bucks from each of the guys.

January 1996

Morris hunches over his black coffee and the "Style" section of the *Post*. They've only been up fifteen minutes and already Linda is cleaning the apartment. She lifts clothes off the backs of chairs and forces them into the swollen closet. She stacks a month's worth of old newspapers and magazines near the door. The garbage can is spilling over. She glares at him as she sorts through rotting left-overs and moldy jars in the refrigerator. They spent the night making love, but as usual, when it's over, they have little to say. She putters around his apartment. He reads. The crazy part of their affair is that she goes home to another man who, she claims, doesn't satisfy her sexually. Her loyalty to this guy is painful for Morris, but Morris can't say no to her. Whenever she calls, they're in bed within an hour.

"You don't have to do that, you know."

"I know, but I can't stand to see you living in this pigsty. How do you expect me to live here? I can't stand the mess."

"Are you reconsidering my offer?"

"Maybe. I don't know. Paul needs me. His divorce is almost final. He may lose his kids."

"Why should I give a goddamn about Paul and his kids? Listen Linda, I can't go on like this. I want to live with you. You've got to choose—either Paul or me. I can't do this anymore."

"Morris, sex isn't everything. Paul loves me. He wants to marry me."

"I might want to marry you . . . someday."

"Might isn't good enough, Morris. Paul is a yes."

He's angry at himself for not feeling certain enough to propose. "I'm not giving you the whole spiel again, Linda. Make up your mind or don't call me anymore."

"Okay." She gathers her things with a sad look that makes him want to take back what he said. Be firm, he tells himself, the line has to be drawn. Tonight he has a date with the beautiful redhead, Ellen. He's waited several months until Mark was out of the picture. This makes it easier to let Linda go.

George bangs on the door while Mo sits on the toilet reading the *Post.* Mo hates being interrupted. "It's open."

George walks in and paces outside the bathroom door. "Mo, guess what I just heard? It's unbelievable. It's awful. A catastrophe."

"Just a minute." Morris flushes the toilet and walks out, annoyed. "What?"

"Billy's sick. He's got AIDS."

"You're kidding!"

"He's gone to his parents in Illinois. Mark told me he's been diagnosed with pneumocystis."

"Mark? How did he know? How could this happen?"

"I don't know. You know Billy, the original wild and crazy guy. Maybe a prostitute or shooting up?"

"He's not a junkie."

"Yeah, but he's experimented. Jesus, we all have."

"I just read an article in the paper that says heterosexuals have almost no risk in this country." He waves the paper in George's face.

"Mo, wise up. Remember those jokes about polymorphous perversity? Maybe he got it from a guy."

"I don't believe that. Bill isn't gay. I've known him since high school. He isn't gay."

"Lots of people are bi. I don't know. Get your ass dressed. Christ, I need a drink."

April 2001

Morris sits in the waiting room of George Washington Hospital. The doctor is deciding whether to admit him or not. His infectious disease specialist says his T-cell ratio has dropped dramatically since they checked it three months ago. He doesn't have any symptoms, but as he digests this news, he begins to feel nauseous. They want him to volunteer for a new drug regimen. There are thirty or more AIDS drugs licensed for human trials. Since none of the vaccines have provided any immunity thus far, the medical effort has turned to early drug treatments. For AIDS carriers, presymptom, pre-illness treatment is common. Unfortunately, most of the new drugs have serious side effects, some of which are fatal. His doctor explains this to him carefully. His head swims; he feels dizzy.

To add to his misery he learned earlier in the day that none of Celia's medical bills will be covered by insurance. He and Ellen will have to sell the house and liquidate their assets to pay them. He doesn't have the heart to tell Ellen. She stays in the house, keeping Celia's room as it was. Her grief has become as solid as a monument. For a few months Ellen tried to continue her practice, but most of her patients quit. Morris wonders how he will pay the rent on his studio apartment. How will Ellen survive without the house?

He thinks of the bills being debated in Congress to subsidize medical expenses for AIDS patients. Three separate bills have been voted down, and the one that passed was vetoed by the president. The Congress agrees on subsidizing some AIDS expenses but disagrees on who would be eligible. The White House says AIDS will bankrupt the government and lead to socialized medicine. A huge clamor has arisen not to raise taxes for AIDS funding. Ironically, Morris is now on the radical fringe and speaks out vociferously for nationalized health care, a proposition he once vigorously opposed. He is frightened by the right-wing religious fanatics and the conservative AMA lobby. AIDS isn't someone else's problem anymore.

AIDS has cost Morris his job. His new job pays a lot less. Insurance companies refuse to insure him and Ellen. What will happen when one of us gets sick? he broods. There's nothing to fall back on except charity. His parents have disowned him. They are convinced he is a closet homosexual. His mother wrote, "Don't come home and expect we'll take care of the mess you've created. How could you do this to that sweet baby?"

"Mr. Apter, come with me, please." The nurse holds out a sympathetic hand. They walk down the long hall to the doctor's office.

"Have you made a decision about the drug treatment, Morris?"

"No."

"We need to start as soon as possible in order to monitor the volunteers over the same time period. Any questions?"

"No."

"What kind of insurance do you have? Some companies do cover this, if that's a concern to you."

"My insurance was cancelled. My daughter died of AIDS, doctor."

"Well, I think you're a good candidate for the no-cost treatment, but the drug dosage will be time-limited. Just fill out a financial statement and bring it back tomorrow."

"How long before I get sick? That's all I want to know."

"There's no way to predict. According to your most recent tests, the immune system is compromised. You could get sick tomorrow or next week or next month. You could continue with minor problems for quite some time. Some of these drugs look very hopeful. They may keep the virus suppressed for a lifetime. We don't know. You could live a normal life, Morris."

Morris laughs out loud. "I could live a normal life." It's amazing what doctors will say to get you into their studies. "My baby is dead. My marriage is ruined. I lost my job. My parents disowned me. I'm bankrupt. I have a terminal disease. And you say I could live a normal life. Very funny, doc." He shakes his head and stares at the floor. "The answer is no. I don't want any experimental treatment. I'll take my chances."

The doctor is not at all chagrined. "That's not a good attitude, Morris. You're not even sick. Think of those who've died. They'd trade places with you. You've got to have hope."

"No thanks, doc. You keep hope. I've had enough." As he leaves, he tosses the financial form into the wastebasket.

In the waiting room Morris sees a vaguely familiar face—Mark Rogers. He's almost bald; his cheeks are hollow and sunken like an old man's. Morris hasn't seen Mark in a few years. George said he moved to Houston. "Hey, Mark? Mark Rogers?"

The strained face turns up, glassy eyes lit with recognition. "Yeah. Hello, Mo." He offers a boney hand, hot with fever.

"What are you doing here? I heard you moved south."

"I did. Lived in Houston a while, but I had to come back. My family's in Bethesda. I . . . I need to live with them." He stutters and seems lost for a moment.

Morris sits down with a thud in the chair next to Mark. He stares at an ashtray full of cigarette butts. "Life's gotten all fucked up, hasn't it?"

"Life, yeah, really. Waiting to die isn't living, Mo. Have hope, they say. We've got to have hope." He shakes his head, disgusted by the idea of hope.

"You don't know, do you?"

"That you and Ellen got married?"

"Yeah. We had a baby, Celia. She died of AIDS."

Mark's head falls forward as if someone shoved it down from behind. His shoulders rise and fall in silent heaves. "There's no mercy." Tears roll over his cheeks.

Morris cringes. He hates what he's seeing. He puts his arm around Mark's shoulders. A long silence embraces them. Morris feels an odd sort of relief. He, who would not be treated or bothered by hope, wants Mark to have hope. "Hey, remember those wild parties we had? Remember the year the Redskins beat Dallas in the Superbowl? Remember George and Billy in the pizza-eating contest? Those were great times."

"Billy. Sure. I was with him when he died." He glances up, his red eyes bulging from the sockets. "Mo, how's Ellen?"

"We've both got it. Celia's death was a terrible blow. We separated shortly after she died."

"I'm so sorry." Mark mumbles. "I'm so sorry." He stands up and leans on his cane, seeming disoriented. "I've got an appointment." He points down the hall. "I knew Ellen . . . " he stammers. "Before she met you." Morris watches him search the room with his feverish eyes, as if the room were his memory bank.

June 2001

The woman in the bed next to hers prays out loud. Ellen stuffs cotton in her ears. She asks for a private room and is told she's lucky to have a bed. She's in the AIDS ward at Washington Hospital Center. Her roommate is close to death, and like it or not, she talks. "My man, that Jamaican. He loved women, that man, but Lord, O Lord, he fell in with them bad ones on the street. They gave him the drugs. I begged him not to. They didn't have no sterile needles them days. We was on welfare. I's a decent, God-fearing woman. I wouldn't go on the streets for no man. God's punishing me now, child. I'm suffering so's to get into heaven. I's repented and ready to go. Lord knows, I's suffered enough on this earth."

Ellen closes her eyes and loses herself in memories. Her mother, sister, and Morris visit her every day. She is being monitored after developing a serious drug side effect. The doctors say they might consider a bone marrow transplant, but this is an extreme measure and the supply of donors is very low. When she first entered the hospital she didn't care what they did, which complicated her treatment.

They tell her the hospital has to make hard choices these days. They want to help her, but they have to reserve expensive treatments for those who stand the best chance of survival. Her body is strong. Her T-cell count is just below the normal range. But her attitude has been poor. She gets the same lecture Morris got. Even the death of her baby doesn't stop them. Too many AIDS cases have hardened them. AIDS has hardened her too.

She remembers the day Morris came to tell her about the insurance and Celia's medical bills. It was a lovely, warm, sunny day. They drank coffee at the kitchen table. She first felt forgiveness that day.

"I ran into Mark Rogers at the hospital. Remember him? He's looking pretty bad. Did you know he has AIDS?"

Her heart seemed to stand still. "No, I didn't." She felt as if someone had hit her with a baseball bat, as if she couldn't breathe. Her face turned pale and she grabbed the table, then fainted and fell forward.

"Ellen!" Morris grabbed her and pulled her back up.

The color slowly returned to her face.

That was a month ago, before she went into the hospital. That day she began to change. She began to want to live for the first time since Celia's death. Now she holds Mark's obituary in her hand, calmly remembering him. No matter how much she studies it, she cannot believe she is responsible for Celia's death. Morris says there is no way to know. They must forgive each other and themselves.

August 2001

Freedom comes to them when they hit bottom. Ellen leaves the hospital and moves into the studio with Morris. Health after a period of illness gives them a new appreciation for every second of life. Ellen's mother has given them some money, and Morris calculates that they have enough money to travel around the world, a dream they once shared but never considered after Celia was born.

Morris collects armloads of books and reads travel stories to her. They dive into history, language and anthropology. They plot a route from the southern hemisphere in winter to the northern hemisphere in summer. They will zigzag from Argentina up through South America to the Carribean, then to the British Isles and Scandinavia, and down through Europe to Africa. As long as they are well and have money they will keep going. Their friends are skeptical, but no one has the heart to question their dream.

While they wait to sell their house and settle their affairs, they calculate expenses and comb travel books for bargains. Sometimes memories surface and anger explodes, reducing one or the other to misery. They take turns apologizing and comforting each other and quickly bounce back from these arguments. Nagging about bad habits is behind them, as are a lot of other worries. They indulge in whatever they want on a menu and never pass up dessert. They make love, something they hadn't been able to do since the day they discovered Celia had AIDS.

The day finally comes when they close on their house and pick up their tickets from the travel agent. First to Puerto Rico, then Antigua. Their friends give them a rip-roaring going-away party. The next day Morris is exhausted. He rests on the only part of the sofabed not covered with clothes and assorted junk. Ellen is packing in a state of panic. For two weeks she has stockpiled the things they might need. She has everything in the medical kit except a spare tire. But she's having a space problem. Four heavy suitcases have to become one and a half. She bites her fingernails trying to figure it out. Morris has his entire life in a gym bag. She picks it up and looks to him for help. "I've got to decide what to leave behind, Mo. I'm getting confused. Can I mail stuff ahead?"

"Just pack one outfit for heat, one for cold, and one for in between. It'll fit in a small bag. Take my word for it."

"Do you think I should take my down jacket?"

"We're never going to be in winter, honey."

"We could hit bad weather."

"For Christ's sake, El. The taxi's going to be here in twenty minutes. The guy renting the apartment is outside ready to move in, and you're still packing."

She moves faster, running in circles, searching through boxes of their possessions for her down jacket. After she finds it she changes her mind. "Mo, I'm hysterical. I can't do this."

"We're doing it. We paid for the tickets. We had our goodbye party and the taxi is on the way. We're blasting off, El." Morris starts to get a case of nerves, too. He double-checks his leather bag for his wallet, their passports, tourist visas, shot records, and traveler's checks. The horn of the taxi startles him.

Ellen grabs her largest bag, gives the apartment a last scan and feels an enormous surge of relief. "Okay, we're off."

Morris deposits the luggage into the trunk and tells the cabby, "Dulles Airport." Ellen looks over the brochure for the Carribean Sun Hotel. In the back of the cab, they squeeze each other's hands and smile like honeymooners. Ellen tries not to think of Celia, but when she does the pain doesn't overwhelm her. Celia's death left an emptiness nothing will ever fill, but she and Morris are alive. They want to live.

The construction of the new Concorde runways at Dulles is in full swing. Traffic is backed up for miles. When they finally pull up to Departures they have only thirty minutes to spare. The luggage check goes speedily, but there's an absurdly long line at security. Morris asks if they can go ahead because their plane is boarding.

"Sure." An elderly man gestures in front of him.

"We have to see your ticket for an international destination, sir."

Morris takes out their tickets and passports and presents them, then walks through the screener. Ellen follows.

"Over here, madam." Another set of uniformed men with F.B.B.I. patches on their pockets sit at a desk. Security is passing all documents to them. Morris reads the insignia on the table cover: National Institute of Health, Federal Bureau of Blood Inspection. He's never heard of them. "Can we see your immunization records?"

Morris opens the yellow booklets and hands them to the balding man. He begins to sweat, his body warning him that something bad is about to happen. Ellen stares helplessly at the men.

"Do you have your blood inspection certificates, sir?"

"What blood inspection certificates? We're going on vacation."

"I'm sorry, sir, but it's a new law. They should have told you when you got your shots. We can't let you on an international flight without a clean blood inspection stamp."

"Listen, buddy, I paid for these tickets. I'm a citizen of the United States, and I can go where I damn well please."

The man signals to his assistant who stands conspicuous in a white lab coat. "You're not going to make this flight, but we can get you on a later one. The tests only take an hour. Just follow this gentleman."

"We're not following anybody."

"Don't you read the newspapers, mister? We're cooperating with the World Health Organization to stop the spread of AIDS. No one without a negative blood test leaves the country. It's the law. If you want to travel, step over there and we'll get you tested."

"This is a violation of our constitutional rights. It's outrageous!" He grabs his papers from the man's hand, grabs Ellen's arm, and they run toward the gate.

The man pushes a small button under the table. Within minutes two burly policemen are holding Morris and Ellen by the arms.

The F.B.B.I. officer shakes his head in dismay. "Looks like they've got something to worry about."

His colleague complains. "I think this procedure is going to get pretty cumbersome. When is the World Movement Procedure Department going to start color coding passports?"

"They've started, but it takes time to invalidate the old ones and mail out renewals," the officer replies.

The line grows longer and other passengers become unruly, complaining and protesting with rising vigor. The old man who let Morris and Ellen go ahead of him is in line at the F.B.B.I. checking station. He catches a glimpse of them being led away to the mobile blood check van. He holds up a sympathetic victory sign, but they don't look back.

PART THREE

Literary AIDS:
The Classroom

Teaching about AIDS and Plagues: A Reading List from the Humanities

"AIDS is a plague." In the early 1980s, this phrase seemed to reflect the journalistic hysteria and community panic regarding HIV-infected people prevalent in media coverage during the early stages of the epidemic. For gay activists, AIDS as plague seemed to be particularly threatening when voiced by homophobic fundamentalists who suggested by this term that infected people had brought the disease upon themselves as God's punishment for their sins. By the late 1980s, as more became known about HIV as a slow-acting retroviral infection, the term "plague" no longer seemed useful, when AIDS, unlike the acute and quickly lethal bubonic plague, became defined as a chronic rather than acute terminal disease.

With the growing epidemic of AIDS in Asia, Africa, and South America in the early 1990s, however, the word "plague" reflected the impotence and sorrow as infection expanded to ever larger segments of populations in nations around the world. As the AIDS epidemic continues to unfold, the word "plague" will take on new meanings. As we cope with the changing face of AIDS, an investigation into the diverse concepts of plagues and how they relate to AIDS both historically and in relationship to modern epidemics may help us gain insight to the ways that cultures, whether they be ancient Greece or modern India, cope with catastrophic infectious disease.

In America, since 1985, the use of the plague image has become central to literary as well as journalistic discussions of AIDS. For some writers, like David Black, in his book *The Plague Years: A Chronicle of AIDS, the Epidemic of Our Times* (Simon and Schuster, 1985) this metaphor evokes historical literary images of epidemics whose emotional power enhances the author's objective depiction of the progress of AIDS. Paul Monette, in his memoir *Borrowed Time* (Harcourt, Brace, Jovanovich, 1988) uses plague images that have evolved from our shared cultural past as a way to humanize AIDS and place its horrors within a historical context. Susan Sontag, in her short treatise *AIDS and Its Metaphors* (Farrar, Straus and Giroux, 1988) uses plague motifs to help analyze our irrational response to this viral disease. Aram Saroyan, in his March 8, 1990, *Los Angeles Times* review of Monette's *Afterlife* (Avon Books, 1990), uses the image to evoke the classical pattern of good men dying young, when he writes about Persons With AIDS: "Their lessons in life accelerated, just as their mortal cycle has been shortened by this new Black Plague." For many literary writers, the term "plague" acts as a cultural shorthand, capturing our sense of sorrow, impotence, horror, and loss.

This urge to make an analogy between the current medical crisis and the Black Death, however, is not new. During past epidemics, physicians and citizens have called various diseases "plagues." Fitzhugh Mullan, in *Plagues and Politics: The Story of the United States Public Health Service* (Basic Books, 1989) explores a variety of epidemics under the rubric of "plague," from Rocky Mountain spotted fever to drug abuse. Charles Rosenberg, in *The Cholera Years* (University of Chicago Press, 1962), and René and Jean Dubos, in *The White Plague* (Rutgers University Press, 1952), show how nineteenth-century epidemic diseases were called "pestilences" and "plagues," while social responses to contagious disease echoed, in many ways, the medieval response to the Black Death.

While these plague images are used primarily because they evoke the horror of mass death, the word "plague" also has the simple dictionary meaning of "an epidemic." Nevertheless, no matter what name we give it, historians of medicine have found that cultures seem to respond in a similar fashion to onslaughts of infectious disease. According to William H. McNeill, in *Plagues and Peoples* (Doubleday, 1976), societies throughout the world attribute lethal epidemics to foreigners or outsiders, exclude infected people from everyday life, and accuse victims of endangering the population at large. In the face of catastrophe, however, we are reluctant to alter established patterns of behavior to prevent disease, whether we live in preliterate tribes or reside in New York City. Hence, the Greek experience of the plague of Athens or the medieval Black Death can be seen as models for more recent epidemics, whether they be cholera, tuberculosis, or AIDS.

Similarly, plague has been viewed throughout history as a physical or medical entity and as a test of moral or spiritual virtue. In the

Bible, in classical Greek literature, during the Renaissance, and into the nineteenth and twentieth centuries, there have been two primary approaches to disease. For some, prayer, repentance, and changes in lifestyle are essential to reestablish one's relationship to one's own body, community, and God. For doctors, governments, and concerned citizens, infectious disease is best controlled by public health measures, usually mandated and provided by the state. Traditional strategies against plague include the quarantine of ships to prevent transmission through infected goods and persons, increased sanitation to ensure clean air and streets, and the employment of physicians, nurses, and assistants to care for the dying and dispose of the dead. Even when the cause and the cure of the disease are unknown, people find tools which they believe might be effective to combat the epidemic.

To best understand what we must do now, we can use the past as a guide, a warning, and a promise of success. The Black Death, or bubonic plague, is now endemic throughout the world, but wild animals, not people, die of the plague. Sanitation, wildlife management, and antibiotics make it a rare disease in humans. The modern plagues of cholera, tuberculosis, yellow fever, syphilis, and polio in most parts of the world are capable of being controlled. Research on AIDS vaccines, drugs to stop viral replication, and treatments for opportunistic infections may help HIV-infected individuals lead longer and more productive lives. If AIDS is a plague, then this image can evoke hope as well as despair.

The purpose of this reading list is to help students understand the historical basis as well as our contemporary response to AIDS. Through an analysis of texts ranging from the Bible and Greek literature to the most recent works on AIDS, students can trace the various ways societies have responded to epidemics, the words they use to describe them, and the strategies they have used to control them.

At UCLA, the course "AIDS and Plagues" is part of a larger educational program available to students. In the graduate School of Public Health and in the biology department there are courses on AIDS in relationship to sexually transmitted disease. The English department has offered courses on gay literature, which includes readings on sexuality and disease. The AIDS Ethics Committee addresses metaphors of AIDS as part of its exploration of ethical issues. And the university sponsors an AIDS-awareness week every year. My course is offered through the Council on Educational Development, which funds interdisciplinary courses outside the purview of departmental curricula.

The class is listed for general upper-division elective credit. The majority of the students have been female, juniors and seniors, with a few honors students, graduates and faculty. Students are self-selected for their interest in literature or health care issues. The readings are extensive, with paperback texts and an anthology of shorter works and medical and popular journal articles which I compile in photocopied form. The students are encouraged to read freely, while specific works are assigned for class discussions. Students write papers, present their research to their peers, and develop a site visit. This visit can include attendance at a cultural event related to AIDS, a visit to a place where HIV-infected people receive support or medical services, meeting with an AIDS activist group, or taking an HIV test for the student herself or himself.

At various times, outside speakers have offered their expertise: a woman living with AIDS, a nurse who runs an AIDS unit in a public hospital, a minister serving AIDS patients, an educator who developed peer training for street drug users, an art historian who compares AIDS themes to depictions of other catastrophes in art, a writer-producer of a television segment on AIDS, and an ethicist who leads the students through an AIDS ethical problem.

Students are also encouraged to check out videotapes of television shows, from dramas like *An Early Frost* to didactic presentations and documentaries found on PBS and cable television stations. Current AIDS news from the popular press are also shared in class. The eclectic nature of the materials allows every student to gain objective information about AIDS as well as have an intense subjective experience of how this epidemic affects individuals, including themselves. The site visit especially brings home to students the reality, the joy, and the sorrow associated with this disease.

In the class discussions, as well as in the readings, speakers, and papers, students are encouraged to gain cognitive knowledge about the material as well as to express their personal feelings, based on their own disciplines and background. I share my perspectives not only as a literary scholar but as a practicing nurse and public health educator.

Based on their experiences in the class and site visits, students have changed their lives. An older male student who organizes parties for businessmen began to question the medical and moral implications of his work. Both gay and straight young men and women have shared their experiences visiting, then volunteering at a hospice. A student who had "never met a gay person in her life" went to a display of the NAMES Quilt and, weeping, held a gay man in her

Soon it owns the body and moves
to the mouth, the holes of secret
access, blows from lip
to lip, dandelion
fluff, invading lover
to lover, mother
to child, the old, even
the dying, no one immune, escaping.
Heart to sinew, skin to bone,
we change in our beds
to things sharp
of vision, long of breath.
There is no cure.

Champaign, IL — *Confronting AIDS through Literature: The Responsibilities of Representation*, edited by Judith Laurence Pastore, combines the work of twenty-three individuals who illustrate the problems and debates surrounding AIDS literature. This growing body of work can be the tool that destroys the prejudices associated with the AIDS epidemic and contributes to a greater understanding of the disease and its victims.

Authors, scholars, and critics review how literature has represented AIDS, address such questions as how explicit depictions should be, and recognize the difficulties of appealing to a public unwilling to face the realities of AIDS. These topics and others are used to establish the responsibilities of AIDS literature. Included in this enlightening anthology is a sampling of contemporary creative writing on AIDS. These poems, short stories, and novel excerpt represent the wealth and variety work in this new genre.

Teachers are using readings from AIDS Literature to enhance courses in humanities, composition and medicine. The final section of *Confronting AIDS through Literature* reveals how three teachers use AIDS literature in the classroom. An extensive annotated bibliography of work in literature, drama, music, television, and film follows. According to Pastore, all work in this list "treats AIDS extensively enough and with enough sympathy and seriousness to make it helpful in combating mistruths about the disease and creating more compassion for those affected by it."

# # #

Confronting AIDS through Literature: The Responsibilities of Representation, edited by Judith Laurence Pastore. University of Illinois Press. September 15, 1993. 267 pp. Paper, ISBN 0-252-06294-9. $12.95. Cloth, ISBN 0-252-01989-X. $39.95.

University of Illinois Press • 54 E. Gregory Dr. • Champaign, IL 61820 • (217) 333-0950 • FAX (217) 244-8082

The University of Illinois Press

is pleased to send you a review copy of

Confronting AIDS through Literature

The Responsibilities of Representation

Edited by Judith Lawrence Pastore

Publication date: September 15, 1993

Price: Cloth, $39.95; Paper, $12.95

We would appreciate two copies of any published review.

UNIVERSITY OF ILLINOIS PRESS
54 East Gregory Drive, Champaign, IL 61820

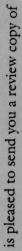

arms. Two young women, terrified by AIDS, visited a home for infants with AIDS and became volunteers. A young woman explored the taboo in her Korean community regarding HIV testing, and decided to work in public health. A young man, as he reviewed his own sexual behavior, became so terrified about taking the test that his site visit became an exploration of his feelings in the parking lot before he ran home. At the end of the course, students who explored various aspects of AIDS in Los Angeles shared their experiences with each other in small groups, validating and integrating their personal experiences into the fabric of the class.

As a result of the course materials and the discussions, the students also develop a critical approach to AIDS data. During one exercise, students analyze policy strategies and their outcomes, recognize the differences between irrational and prudent approaches to AIDS, and consider the most cost-efficient ways to disperse AIDS monies. As future clinicians, voters, and lobbyists, as well as friends, relatives, parents, lovers of persons with AIDS, or as PWAs themselves, these undergraduates develop much stronger tools to help them think and feel about the complex AIDS issues which we confront today.

The reading list that follows was first presented in a workshop I gave in September, 1988, at a University of Connecticut Medical School conference for teachers of medicine and literature. It should be considered a resource for courses on AIDS, as well as a model based on my own experience. Educators who use this guide should alter it at will. The field of medical history and the range of literature written about this epidemic will reveal perspectives on AIDS which were not available when I began teaching this class. Medical historians have begun to investigate epidemics in Central and South America brought by Columbus and subsequent explorers, in the light of AIDS. Educators are developing films and pamphlets directed at specific populations including people of all ages, cultures, races, and sexual behaviors. The news media covers AIDS on a vast international scale, while PWAs and their loved ones will continue to explore their experiences in works of art, novels, stories, poems, theater pieces, and in the popular media. In response to the unfolding story of AIDS, the class should reflect current developments in both the medical and cultural understanding of this disease.

Section 1. Introduction: Plagues, Principles, and Culture

The first section of the class introduces students to the history and principles of epidemics. Excellent historical material is found in

McNeill's *Plagues and Peoples.* Especially pertinent for AIDS are his descriptions of the relationship of plagues to the geographical expansion of societies and routes of transportation and his discussion of the development of cultural norms that protect against disease, as well as the relationship between contagion and behaviors which occur outside social norms. Since disease threatens the very survival of society, plagues evoke suspicion of the outsider and often lead to persecution of scapegoats. For a short reading, use the introduction and chapters 1–2 of McNeill, since students may find the full text overwhelming.

Students also need some rudimentary background in the principles of the epidemiology of epidemic diseases. The teacher, or a guest scientist, can present standard medical information on infectious disease: modes of transmission; problems of the host, the vector and the environment; the stages of the development of exposure, infection, disease, and outcome; different types of prevention strategies; and the ways in which vaccines, immunoenhancement, antibiotics, and other medical strategies can mediate the virulence of disease.

I have found that both historical and modern epidemiological information are helpful at the beginning of the class, but the principles of epidemiology must be repeated several times during the course as new readings cast different perspectives upon epidemic disease.

Readings

Fee, Elizabeth, and Daniel M. Fox. *AIDS: The Burdens of History.* Berkeley: University of California Press, 1988.
McNeill, William H. *Plagues and Peoples.* Garden City, N.Y.: Doubleday, 1976.
Roark, Anne. "Epidemics in History." *Los Angeles Times* 23 Feb. 1986: 10–12.

Resource

Zinsser, Hans. *Rats, Lice and History.* Boston: Little, Brown, 1935.

Section 2. The Greeks and Plagues

The early Greek texts focus on the relationship of plagues to secular and sacred life. In *The Peloponnesian War* (book 2, chapter 5), Thucydides discusses the relationship of plague to war and especially the effect of epidemic disease on the moral and political strength of a culture. In Sophocles's *Oedipus the King,* plague is seen as an expression of violated taboos: it is a punishment from the gods on Jocasta and Laius's disobedience and Oedipus's violation of sacred obligations to the gods. However, in this hierarchical state, the innocent citizens of Thebes become the victims of their ruler's misdeeds. In turn, the king has the responsibility to aid his people and "cure" the plague through his own actions.

In Sophocles's *Philoctetes,* disease does not strike an individual for his own misdeeds, nor is he a scapegoat for his people. Instead, Philoctetes's wounds are part of the larger plans of gods, and he is a victim, innocent of wrongdoing. Nevertheless, his disease contaminates the social and spiritual lives of his fellow warriors, and their leader exiles him to protect them from his impurity. Tormented by pain and isolation, Philoctetes loses all trust in humankind, the gods, and his own sanity.

These Greek texts place plague within a political, social, moral, and psychological context in which societies and governments have the responsibility to care for the sick. When people behave badly, plagues cause further alienation and disrupt social and personal values.

For a short reading, use the opening passages of the two Sophocles plays, particularly those that show how leaders respond to disease. Students who wish to pursue the relationship between disease and sexual aberrations in *Oedipus the King* or the psychopathology of isolation in *Philoctetes* find the complete texts enlightening.

Readings

Sophocles. *Oedipus the King.* Trans. David Grene. Chicago: University of Chicago Press, 1954.

———. *Philoctetes.* Trans. Kenneth McLeish. Cambridge: Cambridge University Press, 1979.

Thucydides. *The Peloponnesian War.* Trans. Rex Warner. Harmondsworth: Penguin Books, 1954.

Section 3. The Bible and Plagues

The Bible, with its complex delineation of the relationship between humanity and God, suggests that God may reveal his power and displeasure through disease and disasters which are often called plagues. Within this moral model, plague challenges humanity's capacity for goodness and offers an opportunity for God to show mercy. In the Old Testament, God demonstrates his force through diseases inflicted on his enemies; plagues are used as a scourge for human wrong-doing, a form of coercion to show unbelievers the power of God's way, and a test of his chosen people's capacity to remain a steadfast in their faith even when faced with overwhelming tragedy and loss.

The Old Testament, as well as later rabbinical texts, teach people through rules for hygiene and behavior how to avoid disease. When illnesses do occur, there are rules for diagnosis, treatment, and the prevention of the spread of infection, including the use of isolation as well as rules for when a diseased person may return to the community. Even lepers, who are separated from other citizens, maintain the rituals and their identity as Jews while residing outside of the community. Within this context of law, homosexual acts are forbidden as violations of rules for living, analogous to other laws that set the standards for diet, hospitality, and reproduction.

In the New Testament, the moral and spiritual treatment of disease is reflected in Christ's mission to heal the people through his power and love. Following this model, people should be compassionate in their treatment of the sick, no matter what their illness. As an expression of the virtue of mercy, men and women have the obligation to offer medical treatment for acute or chronic conditions to all people, regardless of their nationality, faith, or conduct. Similarly, Jesus shows love for all men and women, including lepers and whores.

The story of the Good Samaritan most clearly presents the moral, financial, and humanitarian obligation of citizens to provide short- and long-term care for all sick people, regardless of their culture or background. The readings on leprosy demonstrate both the rational and spiritual approach to healing, and Job offers one model for how to cope with hopeless and untreatable disease.

Readings

Exodus 7–11 (Moses and the plagues of Egypt)
Genesis 19:1–29 (Sodom and Gomorrah, violation of hospitality)
Luke 10:30–37 (the Good Samaritan)
Job
Matthew 5–10 (the Sermon on the Mount and accounts of healing)
Psalms 41, 103 (on sickness)

Recommended

Deuteronomy 12:13–24 (on sanitation)
Leviticus 13:1–15:33 (discussion of leprosy and infectious disease)
Leviticus 18:20–22; 20:13 (man lying with man)
Numbers 12; 21:4–9 (on disease)
Romans 1:26–27 (lust, both homosexual and heterosexual)
Romans 14:14 (definition of "unclean")
II Chronicles 26:11–23 (leprosy)
II Kings 5 (leprosy)

Deuteronomy 23:17; I Kings 14:24; 15:12; 23:7; Job 36:14 (translation of "Gadosh" as "sodomite" vs. "pagan priest")

Matthew 11:8; Luke 7:25, 7:62; Romans 1:26–27 (translation of "Malakoi" as "effeminate" vs. "gutless")

Resource

Spiritual Advisory Committee for APLA. "Biblical Perspectives on AIDS." *AIDS: A Self-Care Manual.* Ed. BettyClare Moffatt et al. Los Angeles: AIDS Project Los Angeles, 1987. 220–224. (on alternative interpretations of Biblical passages on homosexuality)

Section 4. The Black Death

Barbara Tuchman's chapter on the plague in *A Distant Mirror* is excellent for the historical, medical, economic, spiritual, and literary aspects of the Black Death. Of special importance for AIDS is the treatment of Jews as outcasts and as the alleged source of pollution to the community. As a result of these beliefs, Christians treated Jews as scapegoats, seized their property, murdered them, and burned down their homes. Tuchman also portrays the way plague destroys normal social relationships, institutions, class distinctions, and the relationship of the individual to Church and to God. Meanwhile, with the pestilence, death itself becomes a figure of horror, an expression of an irrational and random catastrophe to individuals and to society.

When a historical event is as traumatic as the medieval plague, Hiroshima, and the Holocaust, literature, if there is any at all, is primarily autobiographical. Writings on the Black Death reflect personal experiences, while there are few references in fictional stories or poems. Instead, images of plague abound in the graphic arts: woodcuts and engravings of the grim reaper, the figure of death on his horse, surrounded by corpses, the well caring for the sick, and individual portraits of torment. Similar images of mass extinction and personal horror and pathos recur in art depicting our modern catastrophes, including AIDS.

Among medieval writers, Giovanni Boccaccio's introduction to *The Decameron* introduces the historical experience of bubonic plague into his fiction. A group of young women and men retreat to a secluded estate where they engage in entertainments and pleasures, especially the telling of stories, while the plague rages through their city. Literature becomes a form of therapy, the social act of sharing, while they protect themselves against disease.

Students found the Tuchman chapter indispensable and the Boccaccio material a helpful supplement to her text.

Readings

Boccaccio, Giovanni. "Introduction" (also known as "The First Day"). *The Decameron.* (any translation)

Tuchman, Barbara. "This is the End of the World: The Black Death." *A Distant Mirror.* New York: Alfred A. Knopf, 1978.

Resources

Crimp, Douglas, ed. *AIDS: Cultural Analysis/Cultural Activism* Cambridge, Mass.: The MIT Press, 1988.

Fox, Daniel M., and Diane R. Karp. "Images of Plague: Infectious Disease in the Visual Arts." *AIDS: The Burdens of History.* Ed. Daniel M. Fox and Elizabeth Fee. Berkeley: University of California Press, 1988. 172–89.

Nohl, Johannes. *The Black Death: A Chronicle of the Plague Compiled from Contemporary Sources.* Trans. C. H. Clarke. 1926. London: Unwin Books, 1961.

Ruskin, Cindy. *The Quilt: Stories from the NAMES Project.* New York: Pocket Books, 1988.

Treichler, Paula A. "AIDS, Gender, and Biomedical Discourse: Current Contests for Meaning." *AIDS: The Burdens of History.* Ed. Daniel M. Fox and Elizabeth Fee. Berkeley: University of California Press, 1988, 190–266.

Williman, Daniel, ed. *The Black Death: The Impact of the Fourteenth-Century Plague.* Medieval and Renaissance Texts and Studies 13. Binghamton, N.Y.: Center for Medieval and Early Renaissance Studies, 1982.

Section 5. The Sixteenth and Seventeenth Century: Sexuality and Death

During the sixteenth and seventeenth centuries, disease was seen in terms of individuals rather than groups: the person, rather than the community, experienced suffering. Poets, essayists, and preachers focused on an individual's personal response to disease, dying, and death, as felt by the body, the mind, and the spirit. Disease was not God's punishment, but a way he challenged an individual's faith, while death was a doorway to heaven.

In the late sixteenth century, not only did people suffer from the usual infectious diseases, including brief epidemics of plague, but a new disease affected intimate life: syphilis. Sexuality itself became a source of death. Ironically, sleep was called a "little death," and an English term for orgasm was "to die" with love. Hence, the themes of love, death, the brevity of life, and the ecstasy of relationships became intermingled in Renaissance literary images. Life was fragile, love could be lethal, and to some extent the popularity of the *carpe diem* theme reflected a new kind of urgency. Men and women were advised to seize the day, for life might be short, the time for love brief, and the likelihood of losing one's beloved high. Art itself might offer a kind of immortality to love denied to the actual lovers, and art about love might outlast physical monuments that celebrated mortals' power.

Jonson's anguished lyrics "On My First Son" and his more formal elegy "On My First Daughter," Donne's "Holy Sonnet 10," Shakespeare's "Sonnet 73," and Milton's sonnet "When I Consider How My Light Is Spent" introduce students to the ways men and women respond to disease, dying, and grief. For the *carpe diem* theme, Marvell's "To His Coy Mistress" best demonstrates the power of sexual ecstasy in the face of imminent death.

Readings

DISEASE, DYING, AND DEATH

Bradstreet, Anne. "Before the Birth of One of Her Children."
Daniel, Samuel. "Sonnet 45" ("Care-charmer Sleep, son of the sable Night").
Donne, John. "Holy sonnet #1" ("Thou hast made me, and shall Thy work decay?")
————. "Holy Sonnet #10" ("Death be not proud, though some have calléd thee")
————. "A Valediction: Forbidding Mourning"
————. "Meditations" 1, 4, 14, 17. *Devotions upon Emergent Occasions.*
Herbert, George. "Death."
Jonson, Ben. "On My First Daughter."
————. "On My First Son."
Milton, John. "When I Consider How My Light Is Spent."
Nashe, Thomas. "A Litany in Time of Plague."
Raleigh, Sir Walter. "On the Life of Man."
————. "The Author's Epitaph, Made by Himself."
Shakespeare, William. "Sonnet 73" ("That time of year thou mayest in me behold").
Skelton, John. "Upon a Dead Man's Head."

CARPE DIEM

Campion, Thomas. "My Sweetest Lesbia."
————. "There Is a Garden in Her Face."
Donne, John. "The Bait."
Herrick, Robert. "To the Virgins, to Make Much of Time."
Marlowe, Christopher. "The Passionate Shepherd to His Love."
Marvell, Andrew. "To His Coy Mistress."
Raleigh, Sir Walter. "The Nymph's Reply to the Shepherd."

Resources

The Plague Reconsidered: A New Look at its Origins and Effects in 16th and 17th Century England. Cambridge, U.K.: A Local Population Studies Supplement, 1977.

Slack, Paul. *The Impact of Plague in Tudor and Stuart England.* London: Routledge & Kegan Paul, 1985.

Section 6. Public Health Policy and Plague

Based on four hundred years of recurrent episodes of bubonic plague, societies have developed a series of public health measures to prevent this disease, care for the sick, restrict its spread, and bury the dead. Among these have been sanitation measures, pest houses, quarantine of ships, and, in England, the sequestration of infected families in their homes. During the London plague of 1665, physicians, based on the new skills of scientific observation and assessment, observed that "the shutting of houses," a form of household quarantine, was not an effective method to combat the plague: rather, it only increased the spread of disease and was seen as a form of murder.

When London was threatened with yet another epidemic in the early eighteenth century, Daniel Defoe, journalist and novelist, along with physicians and other writers, reassessed the role of government in regard to bubonic plague. While a wide range of preventive and support services were felt to be prudent and necessary, the concept of involuntary quarantine was attacked in pamphlets and nonfiction prose.

Defoe's major critique of government policy was presented in the form of a novel, *A Journal of the Plague Year.* This was the first presentation of public health policy in a major work of literature and remains one of the finest discussions of the psychological, ethical, economic, and political consequences of government public health measures. In both form and content, it has become a model for other works of literature on plague, including Camus's *The Plague* and Shilts's *And the Band Played On.*

For a short reading on the role of government intervention in epidemics, focus on the opening chapter of Defoe's *Journal* when the plague first enters London, including the Lord Mayor's edicts. Also of interest is the section on spiritual quacks who misdirected citizens with false remedies, the story about the three men who leave London and face discrimination in the countryside, and the narrator's thoughts on the problem of contamination, including the asymptomatic carrier, transmission among family members, and the narrator's analysis of people who seem to deliberately infect others. Students may find Defoe's text as a whole rather difficult and repetitive, but they should respond well to discussions of specific passages and issues.

Reading

Defoe, Daniel. *A Journal of the Plague Year.*

Resources

Leasor, James. *The Plague and the Fire.* New York: Avon Books, 1961.
See resources from section 5.

Section 7. The Moral View of Epidemics

In the nineteenth century, major diseases were perceived in two quite different ways. Infectious conditions were seen as a challenge to the new science of microbiology as researchers attempted to find the specific source of ailments, develop vaccines, and experiment with treatments. Simultaneously, disease was placed within a moral and political context: ill people brought disease upon themselves, voluntarily through their moral flaws or involuntarily as marginal members of society. Epidemics reflected a taint upon a society, whereby sick people were accused of infecting "innocent people." To protect society, whole groups, as defined by race, religion, nationality, socio-economic status, or behavior, should be separated or excluded from aspects of everyday life.

During this period, young adults were especially vulnerable to lethal infectious diseases, including tuberculosis, congenital syphilis, and influenza. During the nineteenth century, early death was idealized and the pale, sickly demeanor of tubercular patients became a model for physical beauty. Ironically, the wasting of AIDS is called "the slim disease" in Africa, and anorexic women are sometimes considered beautiful today.

As Susan Sontag points out in *Illness as Metaphor,* the attribution of symbolic content to disease has disastrous consequences for our cultural perception of medical care. People who have certain "bad" diseases, like cancer and AIDS, evoke terror and are shunned, while people with chronic heart problems or obstetrical complications are treated with compassion and care. Similarly, the image of the doctor as a heroic knight who will win a war against disease is equally mythical, and has distorted our perception of what research and clinical physicians can accomplish, especially with AIDS.

The extensive literature from the nineteenth and early twentieth centuries on medical themes includes many masterpieces frequently taught in standard literature classes. Most deal with early death or the experience of isolation, shame, and depression which are associated with incurable terminal disease. The theme of death and dying is found in Proust, Tolstoy, Keats, Ibsen, Kafka, Shaw, and Mann, and they are appropriate here: Mann's *Magic Mountain* describes the experience of tuberculosis; Kafka's *Metamorphosis* reveals the torment of a son who is abandoned by his family when he becomes physically transformed; Ibsen's *Ghosts* portrays the anguish of inherited syphilis, and his *Enemy of the People* weighs the danger of disease against the denial and economic priorities of government officials.

Sontag's *Illness as Metaphor* offers a theoretical and critical basis for a discussion on the moral and symbolic conception of diseases. For a short list of literary readings, Keats's "Ode on Melancholy" illuminates the poet's personal response to tuberculosis, and Poe's "Masque of the Red Death" and Hawthorne's "Lady Eleanor's Mantle" depict disease as a punishment for immoral behavior.

Readings

Lord Byron. "The Destruction of Sennacherib."
Hawthorne, Nathaniel. "Lady Eleanor's Mantle."
Keats, John. "Ode on Melancholy."
Kipling, Rudyard. "The Last Relief."
Poe, Edgar Allen. "The Masque of the Red Death."
Sontag, Susan. *Illness as Metaphor.* New York: Vintage Books, 1977.

Recommended

Ibsen, Henrik. *Ghosts.*
———. *An Enemy of the People.*
Kafka, Franz. *The Metamorphosis.*
Mann, Thomas. *Death in Venice.*
———. *Dr. Faustus.*
———. *The Magic Mountain.*
Tolstoy, Leo. *The Death of Ivan Ilych.*

Resources

Caldwell, Mark. *The Last Crusade: The War on Consumption, 1862–1954* (New York, Athenium, 1988)
Dubos, René and Jean. *The White Plague: Tuberculosis, Man, and Society* (New Brunswick and London: Rutgers University Press, 1952, 1987)
Durey, Michael, *The Return of the Plague: British Society and the Cholera, 1831–2.* (Dublin: Gill and MacMillan Humanitas Press, 1979)
Powell, J.H. *Bring Out Your Dead: The Great Plague of Yellow Fever in Philadelphia in 1793* (Philadelphia: University of Pennsylvania Press, 1949)
Rosenberg, Charles. *The Cholera Years: The United States in 1832, 1849, and 1866* (Chicago and London: University of Chicago Press, 1962, 1987).

Section 8. Epidemics and Science

In the late nineteenth and early twentieth centuries, with the development of microbiology, vaccines, antitoxins, and antibiotics, infectious disease shifted, at least for physicians and scientists, from a moral issue to an object of technological manipulation. While interventions were possible to prevent or combat epidemics, society often remained ambivalent about the ethics of scientific research and treatment. Paul de Kruif, to educate his audience about the heroic capabilities of the new fields of medical research, created the image of the research scientists, especially the microbiologist, as the new romantic hero. Working in collaboration with Sinclair Lewis, the two writers developed a hero in *Arrowsmith* who inspired generations of young men and women to enter medical fields. In this novel, the complex inter-relationships between private and public life, scientific inquiry versus medical relief for the diseased, and the place of medical work within social, economic, and political constraints are explored. While Defoe evaluated public health policy from the perspective of an informed citizen, Lewis and de Kruif allow the ordinary reader to enter into the thoughts and feelings of the scientist.

For a shorter reading list, the section in *Arrowsmith* on the plague, chapters 32–37, is excellent for the social, political, and interpersonal complications of fighting an epidemic with modern scientific methods. De Kruif's chapters on Reed and Erlich (chapters 11–12) are fascinating depictions of the ethical and procedural problems in pinpointing the specific cause of yellow fever and treatment for syphilis. Students have found de Kruif especially helpful for an understanding of the problems surrounding current research on AIDS vaccines and treatment.

Readings

de Kruif, Paul. *Microbe Hunters.* New York: Harcourt Brace, 1926.
Lewis, Sinclair. *Arrowsmith.* Harcourt, Brace and World, 1925.

Resources

Brandt, Allan M. *No Magic Bullet: A Social History of Venereal Disease in the United States since 1880,* expanded ed. New York: Oxford University Press, 1987.
Mullen, Fitzhugh. *Plague and Politics: The Story of the United States Public Health Service.* New York: Basic Books, 1989.
See resources from section 7.

Section 9. Plague and Modern Society

One of the most haunting images for modern society, with its capacities for technological mastery over nature, is a lethal epidemic that has no prevention, treatment, or cure. Disease again becomes a metaphor, except instead of God it is Nature who punishes us for our hubristic reliance on science and our selfish exploitation of the planet. Plague reminds us of our vulnerability, our humanity, and our need for community.

The possibility of a modern plague as a mass extermination of a people also has roots in contemporary experience: the Holocaust and the Bomb. Just when we thought that our godlike, heroic physicians could use antibiotics, surgery, and radiation to conquer almost any disease, we have seen the destructive capacity of atomic, chemical, and biological warfare. Major killers like cancer could be caused by environmental pollution, personal lifestyles, and insidious, untreatable viral infections. Our society has become aware of the vulnerability of our bodies as well as the fragility of civilization. We have gained a new respect for the powers of disease.

Since World War II, a variety of literary works have used images of plague and epidemics to challenge our complacent belief that we can control nature through science. Before AIDS was recognized, the motif of a major epidemic that could obliterate the achievements of the modern world has been a recurrent theme in modern literature, including horror fiction by Robin Cook and Michael Creighton. The lethal epidemic may appear spontaneously, carried by aliens, or created by a criminal or a mad scientist for his or her own nefarious purposes. Repeating a motif seen since the Middle Ages, the cause of a terrible disease must be a malevolent entity or force.

In keeping with the terror evoked by these fictional plagues, epidemics in popular literature are usually characterized by a very short incubation period, rapid onset, and a gruesome death. In keeping with the myth of the heroic researcher developed by de Kruif, the epidemic is finally controlled through the intelligent strategies of an upright and courageous hero.

Literary writers did not imagine a slow-acting, chronic disease like AIDS, one that infects without warning, remains latent for years, and has no vaccine or treatment. Nor did authors envision a worldwide pandemic, one that has affected people of all races and cultures. When AIDS was first diagnosed in 1981, our concept of epidemics and how to control them was based on myths evoked by recent medical advances and on images in popular literature. Hence, AIDS as a conspiracy, AIDS patients as murderous criminals spreading disease, and hopes for a quick solution to the epidemic were rooted in images already available in popular art.

For other authors, disease and plague raised moral and political issues. Solzhenitsyn's *Cancer Ward* is about politics as much as it is about malignant tumors: it is the corrupt Soviet Union that is diseased. In Camus's *The Plague,* the ordeal of an epidemic of bubonic plague reflects the moral failure of the crass and materialistic town of Oran. However, whether Camus's text is read as an image of the Holocaust, a political and moral commentary, or simply a superb depiction of a town fighting a real plague, he addresses the major medical, economic, political, personal, and spiritual issues of an epidemic. The fight against disease requires moral commitment as much as medical technology. While the plague itself runs its course, the characters recognize their devotion to others and their love for the community, which gives them the strength to go on.

The Plague is indispensable in a study of AIDS and plagues. Novels by Cook and Creighton and a text of Ingmar Bergman's film *The Seventh Seal,* depicting the medieval plague, have historical interest and raise interesting moral issues while they provide light entertainment, even though they lack the power and depth of Camus's work.

Reading

Camus, Albert. *The Plague.*

Recommended

Bergman, Ingmar. *The Seventh Seal.* New York: Simon and Schuster, 1968.
Cook, Robin. *Outbreak.* New York: Berkeley Publishers, 1988.
Creighton, Michael. *The Andromeda Strain.* New York: Dell Publishing Co., 1969.

Section 10. AIDS Literature

Before AIDS, the popular imagination, inspired by the scientific accomplishments of the early part of the century, conceived of infectious disease as short-acting, preventable, treatable, and curable. Diseases that are terminal and chronic, like diabetes, some forms of cancer and heart disease, and a myriad range of debilitating conditions do not have a literature. This lack of images in the arts reflects our own vision of medical care as primarily acute rather than preventive, rehabilitative, or devoted to chronic disease. Neither our doctors nor our society is fascinated by characters with congestive heart failure, metastatic colon cancer, or multiple sclerosis. In America, while there are very moving accounts of childhood illness, especially cancers, we have few works of art that depict slowly dying adults, isolated by their illnesses from ordinary life.

We therefore did not have images available to help us cope with AIDS. Nor has AIDS been amenable to public health measures traditionally used against epidemics. Involuntary quarantine does not make sense, vaccines are not yet available, and treatments thus far are focused on opportunistic infections or prevention of viral replication, but do not cure the disease. Nevertheless, early expectations for the control of AIDS have been based on old myths. We expected that our war against AIDS would result in an early end to the battle.

Meanwhile, the moral concept of plagues has seemed particularly apt, at least for some religious fundamentalists. The association of AIDS with sexuality and substance abuse and the spread of infection among minority groups revitalizes historical perspectives on plagues. AIDS, for some Christians, is a punishment by God for sin. Infected people are shunned like lepers or seen as a threat to the "general population." Groups become scapegoated, while poor, addicted, and ethnic people were excluded from research and treatment. For others, especially the gay community, the stigmata of AIDS are worn with pride, as they engage in political action and develop community resources.

The challenge in literature about AIDS has been to develop a new vision of disease, one that creates heroes out of those who experience disease and those who stand by them. AIDS literature often deals with personal responses to the disease over time: the discovery of disease, moments of personal revelation and joy, the passing of months marked by alterations of function, remissions and relapse, hope and grief.

These are relatively new motifs in American literature and medicine, couched especially in literary structures that best express them. Some authors, like Randy Shilts, become witnesses, using a journalistic form similar to Defoe's *Journal of the Plague Year.* Others, like Monette, use a retrospective memoir. But unlike Camus's *The Plague,* there is no relief from the epidemic, only the loss of dear friends. Work in the theater may focus on personal experiences or include explicitly didactic and political material, challenging the audience not only to be moved, but to act. Most AIDS literature is closely related to autobiographical experiences rather than purely imaginative fiction.

Almost all AIDS literature includes facts about the disease, for its purpose is to educate as well as entertain the public. Commercial television dramas have been active in AIDS education since the late 1980s. *An Early Frost* was an award-winning television movie about a young man who reveals his fatal disease and his gay lifestyle to his conservative family. *As Is* was shown on cable, with its moving depiction of love in all its complexity, as one partner dies. The stories of individuals like Ryan White have been covered in television news and drama, as well as by the press.

Several commercial series have included AIDS issues as part of their plots. Especially memorable is an episode of "Cagney and Lacey" when Lacey, after initial terror that her daughter's preschool admitted an HIV-infected child, learns that casual contact in a school setting would not transmit AIDS. In "21 Jump Street," the young cop assigned to protect a teenage boy with AIDS from his peers discovers the power of compassion when his willingness to touch the desperate young man saves him from suicide. As the characters work out their fears and learn to interact in a humane fashion with HIV-infected people, these television series present both medical information as well as models for humane and responsible behavior.

For some people, popular television shows have become the primary source of AIDS education. News shows with their explicit information, cable presentations of community theater and foreign films, PBS documentaries, and the "AIDS Quarterly" and other recurring series of AIDS issues have brought timely information on AIDS within a global perspective to people's homes. To serve minority communities, health educators are now using popular television formats to provide information. For example, delicate topics such as homosexuality and condom use are raised within a soap-opera format for a Hispanic audience.

Unfortunately, most television shows are not available in script or as commercial videos, and some colleges will not allow privately taped videos to be shown on campus. However, students can watch reruns, colleges can be encouraged to copy shows within legal guidelines, and students can view tapes informally in their homes.

The list of AIDS literary works grows every year. For a short reading, Hoffman's *As Is,* which considers the personal, social, moral, and educational issues surrounding AIDS, has been very well received by students. The performance of the play shown on cable provides a powerful tool to analyze the literary and interpersonal aspects of the work. Its structure is highly experimental, with interweaving plots, time, and fantasies. And, by watching the play in performance, students have found they could better understand how men lovingly interact.

The 1990 film *Longtime Companion* can be used to introduce students to loving social and intimate relationships in gay life. This film also traces a shift in medical care for terminal AIDS patients, from the isolated man dying of pneumonia in an intensive care unit to the partner dying at home, cared for by his lover and a male nurse.

Barbara Peabody's *The Screaming Room*, a powerful depiction of the physical debilitation of AIDS, has helped students understand the process by which HIV infection leads to terminal opportunistic infections and the suffering experienced by an AIDS patient's caregiver. Randy Shilts's *And the Band Played On*, while very long, has fascinated students as a source of information and allows them to critique his particular expectations and bias. Students may also find it valuable to compare Shilts's book to Dominique Lapierre's *Beyond Love*, which provides a European and spiritual perspective on the same historical period. Several students have analyzed AIDS articles in the popular press, especially those in *Newsweek* and *People*, and others have investigated AIDS education in newspapers and advertisements.

Another resource is AIDS art, especially the NAMES Quilt. Cindy Ruskin's book *The Quilt: Stories from the Names Project* and the award winning documentary film *Common Threads* depict not only the quilts themselves but the beauty of rituals surrounding their display, as well as the meaning of their design to the people who made them. Past students found a performance and display of the quilts extremely moving, both as art and as a social experience shared with other members of the audience.

The students in my class, at least initially, felt more comfortable dealing with works that depict AIDS within a heterosexual or political context more than with those that address specifically gay concerns. However, once they became familiar with the themes and values of gay literature, they found gay literature and art especially powerful.

Readings

Hoffman, William. *As Is.* New York: Random House, 1985.

Kramer, Larry. *The Normal Heart.* New York: New American Library, 1985.

Lapierre, Dominique. *Beyond Love.* Trans. Kathryn Spink. New York: Warner Books, 1991.

Peabody, Barbara. *The Screaming Room.* New York: Avon Books, 1986.

Shilts, Randy. *And the Band Played On.* New York: St. Martin's Press, 1987.

Recommended

Monette, Paul. *Afterlife.* New York: Avon Books, 1990.

————. *Borrowed Time.* San Diego: Harcourt, Brace, Jovanovich, 1988.

Sontag, Susan. *AIDS as Metaphor.* New York: Farrar, Straus and Giroux, 1989.

■ SANDRA W. STEPHAN

Literary AIDS in the Composition Class: Teaching Strategies

The "only weapons against AIDS," declared C. Everett Koop in the 1986 *Surgeon General's Report on Acquired Immune Deficiency Syndrome,* are "information and education" (28). Today the epidemic rages with all the intensity forecasted in Koop's early report, and although research continually provides new information, education is still our primary weapon. But the struggle against ignorance about the AIDS crisis and prejudice toward its sufferers has been a difficult one, hampered in large part by attitudes ranging from apathy to disgust, indifference to hostility, irrational fear to a complacent sense of exemption. An important target audience for AIDS education has been—and remains—college students, young people who are just beginning to examine and refine their values, to make long-range plans, to explore new ideas and alternative philosophies and ideologies —and who tend to feel, as most young people do, invulnerable. The freshman composition class offers an ideal forum in which to involve students not only in learning what they need to know about causes, symptoms, testing, and prevention of AIDS but also in examining their own biases and assumptions and the biases and assumptions of their society, exploring the political, social, and ethical dimensions of AIDS as a public health issue, and recognizing their own responsibilities to their communities and to themselves.

The primary objective of the freshman composition class, of course, is to teach students to write effectively, to empower them to express themselves cogently in written language. As composition instructors, we believe that to teach our students to *write* effectively, we must also teach them to *think* critically, to dig in and explore important issues in sophisticated and complex ways. If we want to avoid the kinds of vacuous but well-intentioned essays that examine abortion, capital punishment, gun control, and similar emotionally loaded issues by mouthing platitudes and reciting banal commonplaces, we must encourage students to struggle with real problems and issues, to investigate in depth topics that not only relate to their world but also provoke serious thought about important questions—ethical, philosophical, and moral. The AIDS crisis is a real issue—one that today's students must confront. A unit on AIDS in the composition class can help students explore this crucial subject, learn to ask the right questions, separate fact from myth and rumor, and at the same time provide appropriate material with which they can challenge their thinking skills and exercise their writing skills. The rich and varied body of AIDS literature currently available affords a wealth of material for developing critical thinking skills and for encouraging thoughtful writing—as well as for helping young people learn to make informed decisions, as the epidemic progresses, about personal behavior and public policy.

The topic of AIDS seems a natural for academic research writing—the term paper. Some aspect of AIDS is covered in almost every issue of daily newspapers, weekly news magazines, such popular slicks as *Glamour* and *People,* and every sensationalist tabloid displayed at supermarket checkout counters; statistics abound in the Centers for Disease Control weekly report; and (less frequently, unfortunately) on television, Ted Koppel's "Nightline" occasionally presents opposing views about recent developments in AIDS research or, more likely, about conflicting responses to proposed health legislation. But the standard college research paper may also offer students a means to distance themselves from the frightening realities of AIDS, to collect statistics, cite official sources, quote public health documents, draw pat and sometimes unquestioning conclusions—and still see themselves and their friends as somehow different from all the unnamed and faceless individuals represented by the steadily mounting figures, somehow immune. It is here that literary AIDS can be of immense value. Stories, poems, plays, and essays flesh out the experiences of people with AIDS and of their families and friends, challenging students to perceive them as human beings with feelings, personalities, needs, and interests, as people not unlike themselves, not simply as numbers, wedges of a pie chart, or bars on a graph. The literature of AIDS confronts students with the very personal and complex nature of this human plight, which, in one way or another, will most certainly have an impact on each of their lives. To engage students more effectively in thinking about AIDS and its implications for our society and for their own lives, I use a series of readings, classroom activities, and progressively more complex writing assignments, requiring students to view AIDS from a variety of perspectives, personal, ethical, social, and aesthetic. A sample syllabus, including discussion questions and writing prompts, follows this essay.

In the minds of students, particularly freshmen, AIDS has been so closely associated with marginalized minorities—homosexuals and intravenous drug users—that initial class discussions can often elicit strong expressions of fear, revulsion, and apathy. These attitudes are reflective, for the most part, of the attitudes of students' families, friends, and communities and often serve as barriers to fruitful discussion, barriers more successfully broken down by determined chipping away than by head-on confrontation. To help students move beyond those kinds of "pre-fab" responses and develop more thoughtful and informed attitudes, I have them work through literature that challenges them to examine their values in a number of different ways and that helps them grow to see AIDS as a dilemma of human suffering and death, not as a scourge that affects only those who engage in exotic—and taboo—behavior.

I begin, then, by asking them to examine some of their more general—and often unquestioned—beliefs about the nature of epidemic illness and social responsibility. Poe's "Masque of the Red Death" provides a good starting place and raises many issues that will become increasingly pertinent to students as they engage in the process of evaluating their assumptions. Because the story deals with a fictitious disease in a fictitious setting and unspecified time period, we can begin to examine attitudes without taking on the emotional freight that always accompanies early discussions of AIDS. In Poe's story, the Red Death is so swift, painful, and disfiguring a disease that its victims are refused both aid and sympathy by their fellow citizens. Prince Prospero attempts to escape the Red Death by sequestering himself and "a thousand hale and lighthearted friends" (136) within his walled estate, thus creating in them a sense of security that renders them especially unprepared when the disease ultimately takes them by surprise. Shielded from the pain, grief, and horror suffered by their less fortunate friends and acquaintances, the prince's entourage lives quite opulently until that moment when the revelers, caught in the midst of an extravagant costume ball, come face to face with the uninvited guest—the Red Death. In small group discussions, students are asked to address several questions posed by the story: What are our obligations as citizens and human beings to members of our society who succumb to epidemic illness? What price might we ultimately pay for refusing to face up to the facts of an epidemic, for denying our own vulnerability? And finally, is epidemic illness a judgment on a society or culture, a deserved punishment for unacceptable behavior? These questions touch upon fundamental ethical and personal beliefs; the discussions they generate are lively, often heated, and rarely conclusive, and they establish the foundation for future discussions as the course progresses. The discussions are facilitated by having students keep reading journals in which they record their initial responses to the story and raise any questions they might have about the text. Group activities are essential here, for, as Kenneth Bruffee has pointed out, to encourage students to *want* to challenge the values held by their communities, we must provide them with a transitional community of others who are also willing to make such a challenge (216–17). Peer groups not only create an environment of relative safety for the testing and evaluating of beliefs and values but also serve as support groups as members begin to articulate their new ideas in writing.

Since language is the basic component in writing, composition students should also become aware of the power of words. I have always asked my composition students to examine their own language, and this is particularly important when the terms under consideration are so often muddled or misunderstood. We engage, then, in a close examination of the terms associated with AIDS, what they mean and how they are and have been used. Jan Zita Grover's "AIDS: Key words" is helpful in explaining the important terms, and I use her work in guiding the classroom discussion. It's important to hash out the meaning of AIDS *the syndrome* as opposed to AIDS *the disease,* as it has often been represented in the popular media and understood by the public. Clarification of these terms leads to a discussion of the use of the terms "AIDS virus" to designate HIV infection and "AIDS test" to indicate a procedure that identifies only the presence of the HIV antibody, not the condition known as AIDS. We also look at how the use of such terms as "community" (as in "homosexual community" or the "IV drug–using community") and "general population" (as in "everybody else") has been instrumental in creating false boundaries between the presumed guilty and the presumed innocent (*them* and *us*) and in preventing people from understanding and accepting their responsibility to themselves and to others in the prevention of transmission.

In the AIDS unit, the study of metaphor is a particularly useful enterprise. Here I turn to Susan Sontag's *AIDS and Its Metaphors.* Students are often surprised to discover how many of the terms they associate with AIDS—and with medicine in general—are metaphorical rather than literal. For example, we look at the military metaphor most frequently employed of "fighting" disease by waging "war" against "alien forces" that "invade" the body and "attack" its "defense system" (Sontag, *AIDS* 9–11). Students are so used to thinking about illness in these terms that they have difficulty trying to describe the phenomenon in any other terms. Unpacking the metaphors of AIDS should lead to a discussion of how AIDS itself serves as a metaphor, since it has, from its initial identification in this country, been associated with stigmatized groups and thus becomes a stigma in its own right. I ask the class to think about why people with AIDS prefer to be identified as just that, or even more positively as people *living* with AIDS, rather than as AIDS "victims," and to consider the implications of each of those designations. Students examining the connotations with which AIDS is invested will at once come up with the predictable responses: homosexuality, IV drug use, and death—the three are united in the minds of many students. Rarely are hemophilia, transfusion AIDS, or even infant AIDS suggested in the early discussions, but when these do emerge, we can address the implications of the term "innocent victims." As Sontag notes, where there is innocence, there must be guilt, and we can talk about the problem of blaming the victim.

More recently, the attention of the popular media has focused on cases of AIDS reported to have been acquired through contact with health care professionals such as surgeons and dentists. This introduces a different scapegoat to the AIDS scene: the perpetrator and the care-giver become one and the same, or as Grover puts it, "the innocent are now 'victims of AIDS victims'" (30). Using current newspapers or magazine articles about doctors and dentists with AIDS, the students, working in groups, have been able to discern reporting biases that assign blame and absolution.

Armed with a new sensitivity toward language and a developing awareness of attitudes toward epidemic illness, we next look at an AIDS story, Adam Mars-Jones's short story "Slim." Mars-Jones's story relates the feelings of isolation and depersonalization that the young narrator experiences as he sits alone in his apartment watching his body waste away and his energy wane day by day. In spite of his rapidly weakening condition, the narrator, who is visited regularly by a volunteer buddy provided through the community support group Trust, is remarkably witty, keenly perceptive, and refreshingly self-reflective. Struggling with the loss of identity that accompanies AIDS, he asserts his identity by *refusing* to attach labels. He refuses to name his illness: "I don't use that word. I've heard it enough. . . . I say Slim instead. . . . I have got Slim" (3). And he refuses to name himself: "In Trustspeak, I'm a string of letters which I don't remember except the first one's P and stands for person" (4). His visiting volunteer is identified only as Buddy.

This story is especially effective for the purposes of the composition class because the focus is on the narrator's attempts to cope with his illness and not on his lifestyle or the route of transmission of his illness. This enables students who may otherwise be hindered by homophobic reactions to relate more closely to the narrator's situation—a foot in the door, so to speak, for broadening perspectives and changing attitudes. Group discussions and journal entries concerning this story center on the loss of identity experienced by this extremely person-able narrator as well as the feelings of revulsion, real or imagined, that he senses on the part of his compellingly healthy buddy. Writing assignments ask students to analyze the narrator's central problem from differing points of view: that of the narrator himself and that of the volunteer. Since the narrator is so convincingly characterized, students must deal with him in all his dimensions—his point of view is complex and will not allow any easy answers. Buddy is, of course, a considerably less differentiated character, but students are likely to identify with him more easily because he represents health and is essentially a helper, a good person—he's "one of us." Buddy, the trained volunteer, is careful to hug the narrator, as he has been taught to do, but seems reluctant to eat lunch with him and barely picks at his food. Here students must confront their own fears and feelings about sharing space with a person with AIDS—and frequently their ignorance about the means of transmission. Ironically, they are often quite willing to believe that AIDS can be transmitted by handshakes, utensils, public toilet facilities, and drinking fountains—and frighteningly *un*willing to think that their own behavior or that of their intimate friends could be a much more serious threat to their health. I'm not averse to distributing, or at least reviewing, an AIDS pamphlet at this point, just to make sure they know how the virus is spread—and how it is not. (Pamphlets are readily available from the Red Cross and from state and federal government offices, and many universities now have their own.) A guest speaker can be helpful at this point, someone with firsthand experience with AIDS, such as a hospice worker or a hotline volunteer who can discuss the realities of AIDS from personal experi-ence, rather than a medical expert, who, as Cindy Patton suggests, might reinforce the students' ideas that "scientific facts" will be of more value in their decision-making processes than critical thinking (158–59).

Susan Sontag's story "The Way We Live Now" provides an excellent contrast to "Slim," a quite different slant on the subject, and a dramatic view of people restructuring their lives now that AIDS has touched them intimately. Here again the affliction and the patient are unnamed, but the reader is presented, through multiple perspectives, with the effects of one person's illness on his wide circle of friends. Twenty-five different voices discuss the ailing friend and the progress of his illness. Fraught with varying degrees of optimism and fear, floods of information and misinformation, medical news and home remedies, the group finds itself continuously redefining itself in relation to the patient: "even *we* are all side effects, but we're not bad side effects" (45). And even in their solicitous attention to their ill friend, they recognize that they are "trying to define [themselves] more firmly and irrevocably as the well, those who aren't ill, who aren't going to fall ill, as if what's happened to him couldn't happen to [them]" (45). As the story progresses, certain friends drop out of the inner circle, others become ill themselves, and the remaining faithful continue to discuss the best way to deal with their friend, his illness, and the implications of that illness for their own lives, revealing more about themselves than about the patient. Unable to name the disease themselves, they applaud the ill man's ability do so: "he was willing to say the name of the disease, pronounce it often and easily, as if it were just another word. . . . to utter the name is a sign of health, a sign that one has accepted being who one is, mortal, vulnerable, not exempt, not an exception after all, it's a sign that one is willing, truly willing, to fight for one's life" (46). "And we must say the name, too, and often," one of the speakers adds, but they are never able to do so (46).

Group discussions of Sontag's story center on the attitudes voiced by the various speakers, the thrust of which is that the epidemic has changed the way people—*all* people—must live. Life now requires caution, forethought, restraint in our relationships; it brings a new measure of uncertainty, new demands. The assignment asks students to analyze the reactions of the speakers, deciding, among other things, which responses they could most readily accept, which are most supportive, which ones seem self-centered or counterproductive, and the like, first from the point of view of a member of the circle of friends, and then from the point of view of the patient. This is often an eye-opener because the reactions students are comfortable with as the "friend" do not always serve them as the "patient."

After these writing and reading assignments, students are generally ready to deal with one of the personal AIDS narratives. I recommend

Paul Monette's *Borrowed Time: An AIDS Memoir* or Barbara Peabody's *The Screaming Room,* each of which articulately and eloquently relates the author's ordeal of watching a loved one struggle with AIDS. *Borrowed Time,* the story of the illness and death of Monette's friend Roger Horwitz, is particularly effective for its moving portrayal of a strong and devoted gay relationship, a concept some students have never considered. His chronicle is remarkably honest as he explores his own feelings and reactions while faithfully attending his friend through the long and terrible experience, fighting the frustration of a recalcitrant health care system and a chaotic and often painful—if not debilitating—treatment regime, as well as rejection, fear, and grief. Peabody's impassioned journal records the story of her son Peter and his long, dreadful ordeal. These works not only present true and terrifying portrayals of the progress of AIDS in two courageous individuals, but they also show the strength of the survivors, the friends and family members whose resources have been tested to the limits. Written as testimonies to those who died, both books also serve as clarion calls to action—by the medical profession, by the government, by the public.

Calls to action have, of course, characterized the AIDS crisis from the start and continue to do so. After viewing the NAMES Project videotape *"We Bring A Quilt...,"* I ask students to discuss various ways that AIDS activists have tried to call the attention of the public to the need for legislation, funding, and medical research, to fight discrimination, or to initiate other kinds of change in policy or in attitudes. Recent ACT UP activities are fuel for lively discussions about how the population can be positively—and negatively—motivated. A good collaborative exercise here is to have each group propose an activity designed to promote some aspect of AIDS education. They must decide what audience they want to reach and the most effective method for eliciting the desired response from that audience.

The final writing assignment, based on discussions of the AIDS narratives and their own proposals for action, asks students to embark on a research project that examines a significant change that has come about in public policy, health care, or public attitudes since those stories began. Certainly we are a more aware public than we were; and while changes have been slow to take effect, there have been significant (if not sufficient) improvements in funding for AIDS research, availability of experimental AIDS drugs, and legislation protecting people living with AIDS from discrimination. And there is plenty of relatively up-to-date research material available for students in the form of government documents, medical journal articles, and periodicals whose specific focus is AIDS, as well as news dailies and weeklies and the continuing flow of excellent literary works dealing with issues of AIDS. The difference between this research project and the paper I described at the beginning of this essay is that now the students will have meaningful questions to ask based on their group discussions and their previous reading and writing assignments. They have been confronted in their readings with people with AIDS and with the people who love and care for them, so students can no longer put a comfortable distance between themselves and their research. Working within their peer groups, they should discuss possible avenues of investigation before each decides on a specific focus for his or her paper. Over the course of the term, the group should have developed a supportive attitude toward its members—and a critical voice as well, one that will encourage projects that ask real questions and intercept those that are problematic. Since the group has been interactive from the start of the term, it is important that group members have a chance to share the results of their research projects by giving a brief presentation of their findings to the class; thus all the students will glean benefits from each writer's work, and each student has an opportunity to talk about his or her findings.

For our last few class sessions we focus our discussion on the direction the AIDS epidemic will take in the future. It is clear that now the locus has shifted from the gay community to a more disadvantaged and less vocal one—the minority poor. After weeks of working through the stigma that associates AIDS with gays, trying to expose biases and prejudices, we now begin to examine attitudes toward poor minorities and drug users, an urban population that tends to inspire little sympathy and much prejudice. It is a heterosexual population at that, producing doomed AIDS babies at an alarming daily rate (and at an escalating cost to taxpayers) in New York and other major urban areas. And it is a population rarely represented by literary AIDS, an essential vehicle, as we have seen, for creating public awareness and prompting public action. It is a disfranchised population that has no forum, no voice, either to educate others about its plight or to educate its own for survival. New questions raised by this phase of the epidemic—the distribution of sterile needles by state and local governments, for example—create ethical knots that are not easily untangled and that will continue to demand attention.

I conclude my AIDS unit here—a rather unsettling place to end—with the hope that students who have learned to pose questions and seek answers, examined their prejudices and shared their fears, and gained critical thinking and writing skills through reading, writing, and thoughtful discussion will continue to be actively aware citizens. Their experience with literary AIDS will certainly have challenged their complacency; perhaps it will have put to rest irrational fears; and, better yet, it may have helped replace bigotry with understanding, apathy with compassion, ignorance with responsibility. As the future policy makers and leaders of our communities, these young people will be the ones who must decide, as did Prince Prospero, whether aid and sympathy will be offered to the stricken, whether the privileged will be permitted to withdraw, abrogating their responsibility, and whether the gates of the castle will be tightly secured to obscure the specter of human suffering wrought by the epidemic raging on the other side.

Freshman Composition Syllabus
AIDS Unit

For the next few weeks we will be exploring questions and issues associated with AIDS. During this time you will keep a journal in which you will write responses to assigned readings and class discussions and explore your ideas about the materials we will be covering. Journal entries will serve as starting places for group work and for your longer paper.

Session 1. Introduction: Edgar Allan Poe, "The Masque of the Red Death"
    Questions for discussion and journal entries:
        Was it ethical for the prince to try to escape from the Red Death? In what other ways might he have responded to the epidemic? What were his responsibilities, if any, to the citizens of his country? to his friends? to himself? What would you have done, given the choices, if you were the prince? How would you feel about the prince's decision if you were not invited to seek refuge in his castle? Why do you think the Red Death came to the prince's party?
    Writing assignment:
        Imagine that you are an advisor to Prince Prospero. Write a letter in which you recommend the action that you think the prince should take as the epidemic sweeps across his land. Be sure to provide reasons for your recommendations.

Session 2. Susan Sontag, *Aids and Its Metaphors*
Questions for discussion and journal entries:
What are the implications of using the military metaphor in medicine? In what other ways can we express the idea of a "battle" against disease, the "invasion" of the body by infection, and the employment of "weapons" against illness? How does the military metaphor help us to understand disease? How might it interfere with our understanding? What does AIDS mean? What comes to your mind when you hear that someone has been diagnosed with AIDS? Why do you think people with AIDS want to be called PWAs rather than AIDS "victims"? Why do many people with AIDS choose not to reveal their diagnosis to others?

What is the difference between "risk group" and "risky behavior"? Must one belong to a risk group to be "at risk"? Do you think your physician should be required to take an HIV test? Do you think it is your right to know if your doctor has AIDS? Do you think it is your doctor's right to require his or her patients to be tested for AIDS? Statistics show that many more nurses than physicians and dentists have AIDS; why do you think the public is more concerned about doctors and dentists? Look at the pictures in a recent magazine or newspaper of physicians with AIDS and their patients: how do the photos represent each of the parties?
Writing assignment:
Look through your local newspaper, a weekly news magazine, or another popular publication for a recent feature article on AIDS. What kind of metaphors, if any, does the writer use? Are there any obvious biases evident in the article? To what audience is the article addressed? Write a brief review of the article in which you summarize the main points the writer has made and comment on your observations.

Session 3. Adam Mars-Jones, "Slim"
Questions for discussion and journal entries:
Why doesn't the narrator name his illness? Why don't we know his name? What are his principal concerns? How has his illness changed his life? How is he responding to his situation? How does he feel about Buddy?
Writing assignment:
Write a short essay in which you put yourself in the place of the narrator and describe what your own concerns

would be. What would be the most problematic part of living with the illness for you? How would you feel about yourself and your daily struggles, and about Buddy? How would you change Buddy, if you could, to make his visits more satisfactory to you?

Now think about what it would be like to be Buddy and write a brief essay in which you put yourself in his place. Why have you volunteered to do this kind of work? What do you expect to gain from it? What are the drawbacks? What are your main concerns?

Session 4. U. S. Department of Health and Human Services, "Understanding AIDS"

Questions for discussion and journal entries:

What do you know about AIDS? How is it transmitted? How is it not transmitted? What can you do to prevent the spread of AIDS? Take the quiz "Do You Know Enough to Talk About AIDS?" How did you fare? What is the most recent news report that you have heard or read about AIDS?

This pamphlet was distributed to every household in the United States. What particular issues did the writers have to consider as they prepared to address this diverse audience? Describe the "you" to whom most of the information in the pamphlet is addressed. Can you think of anyone who might not be included in that description? Examine closely the language of the pamphlet; have the writers avoided using judgmental terms? Are the values that inform the statements similar to yours or different? How can you tell?

Writing assignment:

There are twelve photographs included in the pamphlet; why do you think these particular photos were chosen? Write a brief description of each photo and indicate why it was selected for inclusion. Now discuss how the twelve photos work together to create a visual impression designed to accompany and illuminate the material in the text.

Session 5. Susan Sontag, "The Way We Live Now"

Questions for discussion and journal entries:

What different attitudes do the various speakers voice as they discuss their friend's illness? Which of those attitudes seem most supportive to you? Think of yourself as a friend of the ill person; how might you react to his situation? Do any of the speakers reflect the kinds of concerns that you would feel if you were one of his friends? Are there any reactions that seem to you to be uncaring, thoughtless, or selfish? Why might people display such reactions when a friend becomes very ill?

Writing assignment:

We never hear from the patient in this story. Imagine yourself as the person who is ill and describe what your responses would be to the comments and reactions of your circle of friends. Who would you most want to have visit you? Who would you not want to have around? Why?

Session 6. Personal Narratives: Paul Monette, *Borrowed Time: An AIDS Memoir* or Barbara Peabody, *The Screaming Room*

Questions for discussion and journal entries:

What kinds of reactions do you see among the friends of the AIDS patient? How do other people react to the ill person? What attitudes do members of the medical profession exhibit toward the patient? What kinds of support does the patient get, and from whom? What frustrations does the patient experience in coping with the disease? What changes, if any, in the attitudes of the public or in health care do you think have occurred since these stories were written that would have made the patient's experiences less traumatic? How would the stories have been different if the patients had suffered from a terminal disease other than AIDS? How might they have been different if the patients had contracted their illness from blood transfusions? What if they had been poor, urban, minority IV drug users? Should *all* AIDS patients be afforded the same kind of treatment, health care, and funding regardless of how they contracted the illness?

(For an interesting contrast, read Alice Hoffman's novel *At Risk*, the story of a young girl who contracts transfusion AIDS and must deal with the discrimination, isolation, and rejection encountered by people with AIDS.)

Videotape: "We Bring a Quilt..."

Why do you think they decided on a quilt as a memorial? What other kind of memorial might you have suggested? How have action groups such as the NAMES Project changed the way people think about AIDS? What recent activities have you seen in the news media that were intended to draw attention to the needs of AIDS patients or communities at risk? Consider the actions of such groups as ACT UP. Are these activities effective?

Writing assignment:

Imagine that you and your group want to help educate the public on some aspect of the AIDS crisis. You may choose, for example, to try to eliminate discrimination toward people with AIDS, to inform young people about safer sex, to encourage a clean needle program, or to promote a local AIDS support group. As a group, write a proposal for an activity (a demonstration, perhaps, an art exhibit, or a letter to the editor) that will bring your ideas to the attention of the public. In your proposal you should describe your activity and explain why you think it will be effective. Remember that you want to persuade the public to support your ideas and to listen to what you have to say. Be creative!

Final Sessions. Research Project

For this project you will investigate a question that we have touched upon in our readings and class discussions. Select a topic that you have written about in your journal, one that is of special interest to you. For example, if you plan to be a teacher, you may want to explore the policies of your local school district pertaining to children with AIDS or to sex education; if you want to enter the health care profession, you may be interested in knowing what policies have been established for physicians, nurses, hospital workers, and paramedics, who has been responsible for those policies, and how they are carried out; if you are interested in public service, you might study the growing threat of AIDS among the urban poor and discover what is and isn't being done to help; if you are an artist, a writer, or a performer, you might wish to look at the art of AIDS and ask questions about the social responsibilities of art and the artist.

Suggested topics:

School policies for children with AIDS
Distribution of clean syringes to drug users
The politics of AIDS testing

The role of the government
The FDA and AIDS drugs
Medical costs for AIDS patients
AIDS babies—whose responsibility?
Education of the disfranchised
AIDS in the workplace
Discrimination against people with AIDS
AIDS and the health care professions
Women and AIDS
AIDS and art
AIDS research
Sex education in the classroom
AIDS disclosure among patients and health care professionals
AIDS in the Third World

Works Cited

Bruffee, Kenneth. "Thinking and Writing as Social Acts." *Thinking, Reasoning, and Writing.* Ed. Elaine P. Maimon, Barbara F. Nodine, and Finbarr W. O'Connor. New York: Longman, 1989. 213–22.

Grover, Jan Zita. "AIDS: Keywords." *October* 43 (Winter 1987): 17–30. Rpt. in *AIDS: Cultural Analysis, Cultural Activism.* Ed. Douglas Crimp. Cambridge, Mass.: The MIT Press, 1988.

Hoffman, Alice. *At Risk.* New York: G. P. Putnam, 1988.

Mars-Jones, Adam. "Slim." *The Darker Proof: Stories from a Crisis.* By Adam Mars-Jones and Edmund White. London: Faber and Faber, 1987. 1–13.

Monette, Paul. *Borrowed Time: An AIDS Memoir.* New York: Harcourt, Brace, Jovanovich, 1988.

Patton, Cindy. *Inventing AIDS.* New York: Routledge, 1990.

Peabody, Barbara. *The Screaming Room: A Mother's Journal of Her Son's Struggle with AIDS.* New York: Avon, 1987.

Poe, Edgar Allan. "The Masque of the Red Death." *Selected Tales.* Oxford: Oxford University Press, 1987. 136–41.

Sontag, Susan. *AIDS and Its Metaphors.* New York: Farrar, Straus and Giroux, 1989.

———. "The Way We Live Now." *The New Yorker* 24 Nov. 1986: 42–51.

U. S. Department of Health and Human Services. *The Surgeon General's Report on Acquired Immune Deficiency Syndrome.* By C. Everett Koop. Washington, D.C.: Government Printing Office, 1986.

———. *Understanding AIDS.* Washington, D.C.: GPO, 1988.

"We Bring a Quilt . . . ". Videocassette. Dir. David Thompson. The NAMES Project Foundation, 1988. 30 min.

■ JOSEPH CADY

Teaching about AIDS
through Literature
in a Medical School Curriculum

Each fall I teach a half-semester course on "AIDS and Its Literature" to medical students at the University of Rochester as part of the medical school's Medical Humanities program (students are required to take a sequence of two Medical Humanities seminars at the start of their first year and must choose from a list of fourteen to sixteen offerings). In this essay I want to report on my first two "AIDS and Its Literature" seminars, in 1988 and 1989, describing my general concern, purpose, and method and then summarizing my original and revised syllabi.[1] Medical students are, of course, a prime audience for education about AIDS. Unlike older generations of doctors, most of them will be treating AIDS patients at some point in their careers. This fact is nicely capsulized by a remark by a UCLA Medical Center nurse, quoted in Paul Monette's *Borrowed Time:* "If you don't like AIDS," she tells her co-workers, "get out of medicine" (90). It is also clearly supported by projected figures from the Centers for Disease Control: by the end of 1993, when the students from my second seminar will start their residency training, there will have been 390,000–480,000 AIDS diagnoses in the United States and 285,000–340,000 AIDS deaths.[2] Clearly, it is crucial for future physicians to be sensitized to AIDS and its issues.

Like every other major American social institution (including the federal government and the popular media), the medical community for the most part paid little attention to AIDS until the disease started to lose its exclusive association with gay men and began also to be viewed as a threat to heterosexuals.[3] Surely one of the most notable differences between AIDS and past epidemics is that, until a relatively advanced point in the disease's history, the drive for its treatment came overwhelmingly from the population of its sufferers rather than from the population of its presumed healers. There would have been little AIDS care at all early in the epidemic but for organized efforts within the gay community and for the heroic work of some isolated mainstream physicians and of openly gay and lesbian physicians who were willing to take on large AIDS practices. This initial avoidance of AIDS by many physicians is yet another compelling reason for educating medical students about the epidemic. AIDS education might in at least a small way help them to reverse such situations in the future, doing better when they meet AIDS and other, similar challenges in their own practices than the majority of their older colleagues did.

My frame of reference in my "AIDS and Its Literature" courses has been the profound denial that has dominated worldwide cultural reaction to AIDS and that, as such, has inevitably been the context of all AIDS literature as well. My concern was to vivify that problem for my students, so that they might become more aware of its existence around and within them and more sensitive to the need to resist it in their professional and personal lives. Toward that end, I constructed the syllabus around a tension between two kinds of AIDS writing that I have already defined and elaborated on elsewhere (Cady, "Immersive"). The first were "immersive" texts that work to undo the culture's fervent denial of AIDS by thrusting readers into a direct imaginative confrontation with the special horrors of the disease and leaving them to deal with those horrors as best they can, with no relief extended by the author. The second were "counterimmersive" texts that ultimately frame AIDS in some kind of protective way, cushioning the audience (and seemingly the author as well) from too close a contact with its horrors, and in so doing cooperating with, or at least doing nothing profoundly to dislodge, the larger cultural denial of the disease. I assumed that this dialectical arrangement would, paradoxically, give my students a more unsettling experience of the AIDS epidemic than would a syllabus of exclusively immersive materials, demonstrating how pronounced and persistent denial has been throughout the crisis and ideally working better to highlight and discourage any counterimmersive tendencies the students themselves might have.

I chose our readings chiefly from imaginative writing about AIDS. When I did use a few materials that were not traditionally "literary," I treated them as cognitive and imaginative constructions as well as works of information and applied techniques of close reading similar to those used in familiar literary analysis. Of course, this focus and

approach also served my goal of immersiveness. Imaginative literature tends, ipso facto, to be an immersive experience—that is, by
frequently focusing on the individual and on the affective and
passionate, it almost invariably puts us "on the inside" of its subjects
and compels our attention there for a considerable time (unlike other
kinds of writing like, say, advertising or social or political propaganda,
which are interested in keeping us solely on the surface of their texts).
In almost forcing us into close contact with its issues, literature also
becomes a medium in which it is particularly difficult for a writer to
get away with denial, no matter how hard he or she may work to do
so, and this seemingly inherent, general "antidenial" quality makes
literature a multiply-appropriate source for studying a subject like
AIDS, which has had such express cultural denial directed at it.[4] (I
should also mention in passing another major, and more general,
benefit to the use of literature in a medical school curriculum—its
concreteness and affectiveness provide a healthy contrast to the abstrac-
tion and impersonality of much of the scientific education medical
students receive.) To further create a climate of immersiveness in the
course, I ran the meetings fundamentally as discussions; beyond an
opening report on the known facts about AIDS and on the history of
responses to the disease to date, I gave no lectures.

We began the first seminar with the course's most obviously
nonliterary materials: the first article about AIDS to appear in the
New England Journal of Medicine, in the December 10, 1981, issue, and
the accompanying editorial on the subject. The article's primary
author is Dr. Michael S. Gottlieb from UCLA Medical School, one of
the pioneering researchers about the disease and also the chief author
of the first report about AIDS to appear in any medical publication,
in the CDC *Morbidity and Mortality Weekly Report* for the preceding
June 5th. (The name "AIDS," of course, did not appear in this early
material, since it was not coined until July 1982; no distinct term
existed before then for the mysterious phenomenon.) This particular
issue of the *Journal* represented a breakthrough in academic medical
attention to AIDS: all three of its original articles concerned it. This
material is a valuable documentation of medicine's beginning efforts
to understand AIDS and might be of particular interest to a medical
audience like my students, but I used it mainly to illustrate a marked
remoteness within medicine then toward the devastation of the disease.
This detachment may have stemmed in part from the abstractness
and impersonality of the formal medical perspective and of official
medical language, but it also resembles what I would call a counterimmersive distancing from the horror of the subject. The most obvi-

ous example of this appears in the editorial by Dr. David T. Durack of Duke University Medical Center, which is not without feeling for the fearfulness of the situation but is more noteworthy, I think, for its prominent "mad scientist"–like observations. For example, Durack describes the strange opportunistic infections as "a *puzzle* that must be solved" and concludes by saying, "These studies should answer the *tantalizing questions* raised by this new syndrome, *perhaps* providing means to protect the persons most at risk, and *certainly* extending our understanding of host-parasite relations" (1465, 1467; emphases mine).

In our next session we turned to selections from *And the Band Played On: Politics, People, and the AIDS Epidemic* (1987) by Randy Shilts, the openly gay reporter for the *San Francisco Chronicle* who was one of the first journalists assigned to cover AIDS full-time. An extensive tracing of the public and personal dimensions of the AIDS epidemic in America from 1980 to 1987, Shilts's portrait of AIDS differs profoundly from the one in the aforementioned medical articles. *And the Band Played On* has been attacked by some in the scientific and medical establishment for "emotionalism" (Blattner 151), while some gay male readers disliked the book's criticism of a perceived sexual irresponsibility among gay men and its failure to emphasize the heroic voluntarism that came from the gay community in the early years of the crisis. The book can also be faulted for its indulgent and distorting "new journalism" techniques—for example, Shilts's over-schematic and melodramatic use of Gaetan Dugas/"Patient Zero" as an organizing device. But, however one judges Shilts's accomplishment, there is no doubt that *And the Band Played On* is written in the spirit of what I call immersiveness. As its title indicates, the pervasive denial of AIDS throughout our society—by the political establishment, the scientific and medical establishments, even (if there is one) the "gay establishment"—is the book's constant focus. Its extensive detail, developed individual portraits, direct statements of moral judgment and accusation, and blunt use of emotional language, often in the form of relentlessly repeated leitmotifs (some of Shilts's favorites are "Nobody cared," "People weren't listening," and "They waited and waited"), all fix the reader's attention on the outrages in our society's attitudes toward and treatment of AIDS in the first seven years of the epidemic. *And the Band Played On* had been published just a year before I gave my first seminar, and its immediacy was both informative and bracing for my students: it gave them historical information about the epidemic they might not have had before and it stirred feelings of indignation in them parallel to Shilts's own.

Our next reading was a very different kind of text, Susan Sontag's

1986 short story "The Way We Live Now," which was the first fiction about AIDS to appear in the *New Yorker* magazine and, as such, something of a landmark in seeming to signal the literary establishment's endorsement of AIDS as an acceptable subject. "The Way We Live Now" focuses on the responses of a circle of friends to the sickness of one of its members and, though perhaps at first glance daring, ultimately seems a relatively safe experience for its audience. Some remarks that could disturb readers occasionally appear—the person with AIDS is described as "overcome by feelings of hopelessness" (42) and AIDS is called "a catastrophe no one could have imagined" (45)—but the story is dominated by a battery of screening devices that could keep the audience at a comfortable remove from the suffering that occurs. Among the most obvious of these are the facts that AIDS itself is never directly mentioned in the text (the disease is instead referred to via terms like "that" and "it")—and that the person with AIDS is never named (but instead remains a faceless "he" throughout). The dispersed focus of the story increases this distancing effect—the narrative moves from reaction to reaction among the group of friends (who also are barely individuated and are identified by first name only), with the person with AIDS himself frequently hidden from view. The narrator's tone also permits the option of remoteness—not even a member of the group of friends, he or she is instead an omniscient outsider who speaks in the cool and detached tone of a reporter (one of the narrator's typical remarks about the person with AIDS is "he's reported to have said" [47]).

Of course, the point of "The Way We Live Now" might be precisely to criticize the detachment it amply illustrates—for example, Sontag has one of the friends accuse the others of being "cool and rational" about the situation (46). But one can still wonder why, at a time of rapidly mounting cases and a continuing struggle to gain attention and services for the disease, Sontag chose to make detachment the dominant focus of her text rather than to attack that defense in her audience by an unrelieved presentation of the devastation of AIDS itself.[5] In this respect, "The Way We Live Now" seems to me a prime example of counterimmersive AIDS writing. In the seminar it provided an excellent counterpoint to the preceding impassioned work by Shilts, and I hoped it would generate a mounting uneasiness in my students as they saw from it how widespread in our culture the preference for a distancing and self-protecting stance toward AIDS might be. (In addition to having the imprimatur of the prestigious *New Yorker*, Sontag's prototypical counterimmersive text was later selected for inclusion in *The Best American Short Stories 1987*.)

Our next readings were selections from Paul Monette's 1988 book of poems *Love Alone* and his accompanying prose memoir of the same year, *Borrowed Time*, which focus on the suffering and death of Monette's lover, Roger Horwitz, from AIDS in 1986 and which were, in effect, the centerpieces of the seminar. Both books, but especially the poems, are masterpieces of immersive AIDS writing; they are the texts I would recommend most if one had to limit one's teaching about AIDS to a single writer's work. In his preface to *Love Alone*, Monette says that he wants to "allow" his audience "no escape" from the horrors of AIDS (xii), which he accomplishes masterfully in the poems through both content and form. *Love Alone* is dominated by direct, explicit, and extreme statements of painful personal feeling (for example, Monette presents himself as "howling," "fuming," "sobbing," "shrieking," "burning," "aching," and "screaming" at his loss of Rog—[16, 20, 23, 32, 38, 39, 56]), and the poems' relentlessly "chaotic" form perfectly parallels this experience of devastation. For instance, each poem contains striking variations in reference, focus, and tone. They move—and sometimes jump—back and forth in time and from subject to subject in the present and they can shift from piercing painfulness to camp humor to bitter sarcasm to heartfelt pathos and compassion in the course of one work. Fittingly, Monette strips each poem of conventional structure, syntax, and style, as if these traditional markers would be too stabilizing for the turbulent story he has to tell. For example, no poem contains stanza breaks, punctuation, or extra spacing between sentences; each moves from first word to last in a single, long block. Furthermore, no capital letters are used except for proper names and the italicizing of certain phrases for emphasis. In addition, the overwhelming majority of lines are run-on rather than end-stopped.

In one of the poems in *Love Alone* Monette describes his soul as "smashed to bits" by his loss of Rog and by his experiences during his lover's suffering and death (24); and his relentlessly disruptive approach in the book is at once a piercing representation of that devastation and an effort to "smash" his readers as well—to make them feel as shattered as everyone affected by AIDS has been at times and also to impress upon them the special senses of havoc and isolation gay men felt at the beginning of the crisis, when they were left almost entirely to their own resources to deal with the frightening and baffling disease. *Borrowed Time* treats the same general experience as *Love Alone* but with the greater detail and development allowed by a long prose work. As a relatively linear narrative conforming to accepted rules of syntax, structure, and typography, *Borrowed Time* should be more immediately accessible to readers than *Love Alone*. However, as if aware that these qualities might undermine the unnerving of the reader that he clearly feels must be central to any writing about AIDS, Monette freely departs from straight-line narration (e.g., shifting from narration to personal or political testimony), and he is as emphatically intense and emotional in *Borrowed Time* as he is in *Love Alone*. The relentless immersiveness of both books contrasted forcefully with the preceding, controlled and cool Sontag text, and my students found them extremely moving and markedly discomfiting.

After these persistently confronting materials, I ended the first seminar with selections from a work that suggested how tenacious and subtle the cultural avoidance I was highlighting in the course could be. This was Alice Hoffman's *At Risk* (1988), a novel about an eleven-year-old "All-American" suburban girl who contracts AIDS from a blood transfusion. At times unbearably wrenching, *At Risk* might at first seem to be a bridging work, an attempt to make AIDS less of a "foreign" reality for mainstream readers by showing that it can affect them as well as the minority groups more popularly associated with the disease. Yet there is such an objective discrepancy between the epidemiology of the disease and the situation highlighted in *At Risk* that one wonders whether Hoffman is actually working on a more muted and perhaps unconscious level to reassure the mainstream audience and let it maintain its protective distance from AIDS. She disengages AIDS from the unnerving realities of homosexuality and IV drug use, placing AIDS in a situation that actually represents a minuscule proportion of the disease's epidemiology. (Most pediatric AIDS cases are poor infants of color who contract the disease in utero; furthermore, at the time of *At Risk*'s publication, only 13 percent of pediatric AIDS cases resulted from blood transfusions and only 0.2 percent of all pediatric AIDS cases were girls of the central character's age).[6]

Indeed, the amount of popular attention given to *At Risk* at its publication seems ironic confirmation of the book's relative safety for general readers. The novel was a main selection of the Book-of-the-Month Club, and within two weeks of its appearance it was reviewed in both the daily and Sunday *New York Times* (Lehmann-Haupt; Shephard) and an interview with the author appeared in the daily *Times* (James). In contrast, Paul Monette's more uncomfortable *Borrowed Time*, which appeared almost simultaneously with *At Risk*, was never discussed in the daily *Times* and not reviewed in the Sunday *Times Book Review* until three months after publication (W. Hoffman). By thus ending the seminar with a further and less obvious suggestion of the denial we had been investigating rather than with a ringing and consoling resolution to it, I hoped to discourage my students from feeling that they now had all the issues of the course under control. I wanted to leave them instead with an edge of uneasiness that might keep them in greater attentiveness and readiness about the problems in society and medical care that the AIDS epidemic highlights.

When I taught the course again the next year, I worked to keep its essential concern and spirit, though I made some significant changes in the syllabus (and because the course had now been lengthened a week, I had time for more materials as well). For the most part, the changes were in response to student reactions to some of the earlier readings and to requests some of them made on their evaluations for more materials from or about other risk groups.[7] Though they did not say so directly, by the latter comment the students obviously meant groups other than gay men, since homosexuals had overwhelmingly been the focus of our previous readings. In responding to this request, I proceeded with great care. As indicated by the jump in social attention to AIDS once it began to be perceived as a threat to heterosexuals, the aversion that our society first showed to the disease had almost everything to do with the fact that the already stigmatized gay male community was the group first struck in full force by AIDS. A special double denial resulted from the fact that a particularly horrible and seemingly ungovernable medical condition hit a minority group long classed as uniquely unspeakable to begin with—that is, a disease frightful enough in itself immediately became doubly unthinkable because of its apparently exclusive association with a group whose existence and worth society had long denied in the first place.[8] Painful jokes that circulated early in the epidemic, such as the claim that if AIDS had been a disease of Catholic cardinals or Wall Street investment bankers the cure would have been found within a month, were experienced as all too true by the gay community. To observers of the shifting public attention to the disease it almost seemed that the media, government, and other institutions were *glad* to see AIDS emerging in other groups such as hemophiliacs and IV drug users, so that they would no longer have to think and talk so much about homosexuals.[9]

Substantially shifting the focus of our readings away from homosexuality thus ran the risk of cooperating not only with homophobia but with the denial I was trying to dislodge in the course in the first place, since homophobia played such a crucial role in producing our society's initial large-scale avoidance of AIDS. Fortunately, I was helped in resolving this dilemma by the epidemiological facts of the disease and by the shape that AIDS literature has taken so far. Though statistics now show a greater proportional rise in infectivity in other risk groups (heterosexuals, IV drug users, and children), in absolute numbers gay men remain by far the largest group of diagnosed AIDS cases in the United States, and AIDS literature so far has overwhelmingly been by or about gay men. When compared with gay men, the newer, faster-growing AIDS populations have, for whatever reasons, barely written yet about their experiences of the disease.[10] As I shall illustrate, I was able to include some significant new readings by or about other risk groups. But because of the facts just mentioned, I could show that such materials were still not often separable from homosexuality and, in so doing, I could implicitly address and seek to check any homophobic feelings my students still might have.

The changes I made in the syllabus in the first part of the course maintained the dialectic between immersive and counterimmersive portrayals of AIDS from the previous year but with what I hoped would be an intensifying of its tensions. To our opening medical readings I added a more recent *New England Journal* piece, from the September 7, 1989 issue. This was an essay called "When a House Officer Gets AIDS" by Dr. Hacib Aoun, who contracted the virus in a workplace accident in early 1983, while a resident at Johns Hopkins (a capillary tube containing the blood of an infected patient shattered as he tried to seal it, lacerating his finger). Rare as one of the few writings by a heterosexual male with AIDS, this essay was meant in part to meet the students' desire for materials from other groups, but I emphasized even more its sharp contrast with the accompanying medical readings and its implicit illustration of the situation denounced by critics like Shilts. For example, the addition of Aoun's essay brought an immersive text right up against the counterimmersive medical writings from the first class, showing us a physician painfully *in* the situation discussed with such detachment by other physicians. Especially pertinent here, and potentially very discomfiting for my students, was Aoun's description of being shunned by his colleagues after his diagnosis: "Only a handful of people from the medical community came forward to help us," he states (695). The aversion shown by his fellow physicians seemed to verify the point about pathological scientific remoteness that I drew from the other medical articles. It was also a vivid confirmation from within the medical profession of one of the major points made about it in *And the Band Played On;* and since their relevance was even more obvious now by juxtaposition to our other materials, I kept the same earlier Shilts readings for our second week.

For the third meeting I added to the Sontag text a 1988 story called "Slim" by the British gay writer Adam Mars-Jones, about a gay man with AIDS in London. "Slim" is narrated by the protagonist and shows a tightly controlled PWA who works to maintain a strict distance from the painfulness of his situation, forbidding any expression of what the story calls "distressing information" and, like the Sontag tale, even excluding any mention of the word "AIDS" itself (1). Here the banishment is openly admitted; as the story begins, the narrator announces that he has taken "that word . . . out of circulation," at least in his private world, opting instead for the more euphemistic term of the title, the label by which AIDS is colloquially known in Africa (1). The addition of "Slim" to this part of the syllabus increased the tension between immersive and counterimmersive outlooks in the course. Side by side with the Sontag text, the Mars-Jones story suggested how widespread and inviting counterimmersiveness could be—here many of the same distancing features evident in Sontag's work appeared, even in a tale about a frankly gay PWA by an openly gay male writer.

I kept the same Monette readings for the next meeting, as might be expected, but made substantial changes in the remainder of the course. First, I dropped Hoffman's *At Risk* from the syllabus. In the previous year the students' feelings about the novel had been overwhelmingly negative, and they were so quick to pick up its subtly diversionary and placating strategies that there seemed no point in spending precious class time on the book again. So for our last two weeks I substituted readings from two other works: Barbara Peabody's 1986 *The Screaming Room: A Mother's Journal of Her Son's Struggle with AIDS* and George Whitmore's 1988 *Someone Was Here: Profiles in the AIDS Epidemic.* These books are either by or about other risk groups, but also fit the situation described above in still not being separable from homosexuality. They thus allowed me to meet that concern from the students, while at the same time checking any homophobia that might underlie it. Both works were also in different ways immersive, and I realized that by ending now with an exclusive focus on the immersive I chanced losing the frustrating discomfort I had hoped to instill in the students with my previous dialectical arrangement of readings. My hope now was that they would be made equally, if not identically, uneasy by the painful realities this other material sought to confront them with directly.

The Screaming Room chronicles Barbara Peabody's experience caring for her son, Peter Vom Lehn, between his diagnosis with AIDS in

December 1983 and his death the following November. The first extended instance of what would become a notable body of American writing about AIDS caregiving, the book presents a heterosexual woman writing for an audience of people much like herself and understandably devotes considerable time to her own struggle and anguish in the situation.[11] However, anyone hoping that *The Screaming Room* will relieve him or her from thinking about homosexuality will be disappointed, for, as the subtitle makes clear, the book's major focus, and indeed its entire reason for being, is the suffering and death of Peabody's son—and he, reflecting the disease's predominant epidemiology, is gay. At times, *The Screaming Room* is achingly moving. Like Paul Monette, and as indicated by her title, Peabody is not at all ashamed to be frankly emotional. By her detailed depiction of Peter's disintegration and death (he had a particularly virulent course of the disease, with thrush, herpes, diarrhea, TB, cytomegalovirus, blindness, toxoplasmosis, and pneumocystis carinii pneumonia), she persistently engages us in the cruel devastation of AIDS and also vehemently protests the discrimination Peter and other gay PWAs experience simply because they are homosexual. In comparison with Monette's work, however, *The Screaming Room* is less pervasively immersive; by following a relatively conventional narrative line and frequently casting the story as a family drama, Peabody gives her audience anchors that Monette's relentless disruptiveness does not. I suggested to the class that this difference might stem from Peabody's inevitable heterosexual privilege—no matter how harrowed she and others in her situation may be by their contact with AIDS, the cultural support and status she still enjoys as a heterosexual might make her world seem less thoroughly shattered than that of a gay person in the same situation, who would already have been battered by his or her prior stigma as outcast and sub-human before having to deal with the added assault of AIDS.

George Whitmore's *Someone Was Here* is a journalistic profile of three different people and communities with AIDS. The book's final section, a portrait of the AIDS team and AIDS patients at Lincoln Hospital in the South Bronx, based on Whitmore's month-long observation of the AIDS service at Lincoln in February 1987, is the only detailed portrait so far in AIDS literature of the IV drug–using AIDS population, most of whom are poor, black or Hispanic, and heterosexual. I assigned this portion of *Someone Was Here* for our last class, as a rare imaginative picture of this fast-growing and second-largest AIDS risk group in the United States. Yet here, too, the material was not separable from homosexuality, though in a different way from

Peabody's book. In this case it was the author who was gay and, furthermore, a person with AIDS (Whitmore died in April 1989). This situation indicated another sense in which gay men have thus far been central to writing about AIDS—though the devastated out-siders Whitmore describes in his portrait of Lincoln Hospital include few homosexuals, his book suggested that the only people willing to write in detail about this other large group of AIDS sufferers, at least up until that time, were the other afflicted outsiders in the AIDS population, gay men. Whitmore's immersiveness in *Someone Was Here* is of a markedly different kind from the other authors discussed, though arguably no less effective. He works more by an understated accumulation of fact and detail than by the raw cries from the heart we hear in Monette and Peabody, recording in a documentary-like style the daily frustration and burnout of the medical and social service team and heartbreaking incidents like the death of Federico, a two-and-a-half-year-old with cerebral palsy who contracted the virus in utero and who had been living in the hospital because there was no one left to take care of him (besides an aging and unwell grand-uncle) after both his parents died from AIDS.

This course seemed to work well. I had maximum enrollments in both seminars, and the student evaluations included remarks like the following, which confirmed my hunch about the preconceptions of some students and substantiated my decision to structure the course chiefly in a "disturbing" dialectical way: "The assigned readings were informative as well as thought-provoking. I can honestly say that I was forced to face various homophobic stereotypes which I possessed but adamantly denied"; "This course allowed me to explore personal biases that stem from subtle fears"; "I really enjoyed being exposed to the feelings of people with AIDS. That was a world I was not familiar with. The literature examples were broad enough to give many perspectives (i.e., medical journals to poems). I really learned quite a bit, but, more importantly, it made me *think!*" Of course, the medical setting in which I give this course has its special concerns and limitations. My opening medical readings, for instance, might have less interest and usefulness for a more general student audience. In addition, the half-semester length clearly restricted the number of works I could assign, and this problem was only compounded by the press of the basic science courses my students were taking at the same time, which forced me to excerpt the longer texts rather than assign them whole or in long, self-contained sections.

The same condition made me limit my coverage to the risk groups with the largest percentage of AIDS cases nationwide and would make it hard to change the syllabus in the future without sacrifice. For example, I see that any subsequent seminars will have to have some representation of women with AIDS. Though at present women with AIDS make up a relatively small proportion of cases in absolute numbers, and though very few of them have yet published anything about their experience of AIDS, the greatest proportional rise in new U.S. AIDS cases is occurring among them (in the "heterosexual contact" category), and for that reason they clearly should be included in future seminars.[12] Yet because of time constraints, that change can only be made by eliminating some existing readings. To compensate for such inevitable limitations, I distribute to the students a supplementary annotated bibliography of all the significant AIDS writing in book form that I know of, including what might usually be thought of as "secondary sources," such as historical studies and books on psychological counseling and law. Though my "AIDS and Its Literature" course was developed for a medical audience, I believe its basic emphasis and approach are adaptable to any teaching situation. Until social, political, and medical attitudes change, I would recommend organizing any nonlaboratory course about AIDS around the problem of denial and around the immersive and counterimmersive texts that have been authors' deliberate or inadvertent responses to that problem. For the reasons stated earlier, I believe literature is a particularly useful tool for countering that powerful denial, even when, as in the case of counterimmersive AIDS writing, what literature may chiefly impress upon us is the uncomfortable possibility that our culture profoundly wishes not to face the subject of AIDS at all.

Notes

Portions of this article were first delivered in a paper at the 1989 annual convention of the International Society for AIDS Education and in a lecture in the History of Medicine Lecture Series at the Albert Einstein College of Medicine. I am grateful to the ISAE and to Steven C. Martin, M.D., of Einstein for inviting me to speak. Thanks also to audience members on those occasions for useful comments.

1. My discussion here is limited to the two courses I had taught at the time this essay was first drafted (summer 1990) and to the materials available at the times of those courses. Between then and this final revision (summer 1991), I have given one more seminar and am about to start a fourth. My general goals and method have remained the same in these later courses, though I have made a few changes in the readings. I would be happy to share my later syllabi with readers upon request. Address correspondence about this (and about the bibliography I men-

tion later) to me at the Division of the Medical Humanities, Box 676, University of Rochester Medical School, Rochester, NY 14642.

2. Unless otherwise indicated, the epidemiological information in this essay is based on the AIDS Monthly Surveillance Report of the U.S. Centers for Disease Control; percentages are my own calculations from CDC figures. The figures mentioned here are from the July 1991 report.

3. The jump in social and medical attention to AIDS once the disease began to be recognized as a threat to heterosexuals started in early 1985, after the appearance of the first newspaper stories about AIDS among female prostitutes. For a discussion of that shift and of the homophobia underlying it, see Shilts 508–13.

4. In holding here that literature can have or promote a kind of faithfulness to experience, I clearly dissent from the powerful "theory" movement in current literary studies. At its extremes, this outlook portrays literature as an actively lying medium—with its insistence, for example, on the "duplicity that literary theory has increasingly identified as inherent in the operations of language" (Edelman 302)—and seems suffused by hatred for it. I put "theory" in quotation marks because I share John M. Ellis's view that literary poststructuralism is not a theory at all, in that it precludes itself from being analyzed and tested on evidentiary grounds (153–59).

5. For more on my points about Sontag here, and about Monette and Mars-Jones later, see Cady, "Immersive."

6. I base these calculations on the figures in Heyward and Curran. Hoffman does include a gay PWA as a secondary character in *At Risk,* a man whom the girl's father befriends after getting help from him on an AIDS hotline. However, Hoffman told a *New York Times* reporter that her first reaction was to leave the character out of the book and that she only restored him when a friend with AIDS told her that without him the book would be "completely divorced from social reality" (James).

7. In AIDS education it is more accepted now, as well as more accurate, to refer to "risk behaviors" for AIDS rather than to AIDS "risk groups." But I retain that earlier terminology because almost all writing about AIDS does, de facto, focus on particular groups with the disease. In addition, the CDC still classifies epidemiological information in those terms.

8. For more on this cultural situation, see Cady, "Immersive"; for more on the history of these particular stigmas about homosexuality, see Cady, "Teaching."

9. Consider, for example, the fact that the landmark May 1990 federal legislation approving emergency funds for AIDS care was named the "Ryan White Bill". Consider, too, Representative John Lewis's remark on that occasion: "There is no way we can go around anymore saying this is an issue just affecting the gay community. In recent days, the life and death of Ryan White brought it home to many, many people" (Rasky).

10. A comparison of CDC figures for August 1990 with those for July 1991 (the latest report available as of the final revision of this article) shows that the U.S. group with the greatest proportional rise in new AIDS cases was the "heterosexual contact" category, with a 27.83 percent increase, and, within that, a 28.73 percent

rise among heterosexual women. Next was the "undetermined adult" category, with a 25.37 percent increase. Third were IV drug users, with a 23.69 percent increase in new cases. This was followed by the category of children with a parent who has AIDS or is at risk for the disease, with a 22.41 percent rise. Gay and bisexual men, in contrast, had a 20.21 percent rise in new cases, a percentage point behind the 21.48 percent rise in new cases nationwide. However, when seen in absolute numbers the situation for the same period is much different. Gay and bisexual men still make up by far the largest group of diagnosed AIDS cases in the United States, with 64.30 percent of the national total. This is followed by IV-drug users, at 21.82 percent. "Heterosexual contact" cases constitute just 5.5 percent of the national total, and heterosexual women, 3.32 percent. The "undetermined adult" category has 3.65 percent of cases nationwide, and children with a parent who has AIDS or is at risk for the disease make up 1.44 percent of the national total.

11. Other notable examples of this literature of AIDS caregiving are Pearson, Monette (*Borrowed Time*), the relevant essays in Rieder and Ruppelt, and Cox.

12. As of the July 1991 CDC report, women with AIDS were 9.98 percent of the national total, with women who contracted HIV through IV drug use making up 5.08 percent of the total and women who contracted HIV through heterosexual contact at 3.32 percent of the total. As indicated in note 10, however, the greatest proportional rise in new cases nationwide is among women in the "heterosexual contact" category, at 28.73 percent, and the proportional increase for women who contracted HIV through IV drug use is not far behind, at 25.50 percent. One of the few examples of writing by HIV-infected women is the "Women with AIDS/ARC and HIV-positive Women" section of Rieder and Ruppelt.

Works Cited

Aoun, Hacib. "When a House Officer Gets Aids." *New England Journal of Medicine* 321 (1989): 693–96.

Best American Short Stories 1987. Ed. Ann Beattie, with Shannon Ravenel. Boston: Houghton Mifflin Co., 1987.

Blattner, William A. Review of *And the Band Played On*, by Randy Shilts. *Scientific American* Oct. 1988: 148–51.

Cady, Joseph. "Immersive and Counterimmersive Writing about AIDS: The Achievement of Paul Monette's *Love Alone.*" *Writing AIDS.* Ed. Timothy F. Murphy and Suzanne Poirier. New York: Columbia University Press, 1993.

———. "Teaching Homosexual Literature as a 'Subversive' Act." *Journal of Homosexuality* 24 (forthcoming).

Cox, Elizabeth. *Thanksgiving: An AIDS Journal.* New York: Harper and Row, 1990.

Durack, David T. "Opportunistic Infections and Kaposi's Sarcoma in Homosexual Men." *New England Journal of Medicine* 305 (1981): 1465–67.

Edelman, Lee. "The Plague of Discourse: Politics, Literary Theory, and AIDS." *South Atlantic Quarterly* 88 (1989): 301–17.

Ellis, John M. *Against Deconstruction*. Princeton: Princeton University Press, 1989.

Gottlieb, Michael S., et al. "*Pneumocystis carinii* Pneumonia and Mucosal Candidiasis in Previously Healthy Homosexual Men: Evidence of a New Acquired Cellular Immunodeficiency." *New England Journal of Medicine* 305 (1981): 1425–31.

———. "*Pneumocystis* Pneumonia—Los Angeles." *Morbidity and Mortality Weekly Report* 5 June 1981: 250–52.

Heyward, William L., and James W. Curran. "The Epidemiology of AIDS in the U.S." *Scientific American* Oct. 1988: 72–81.

Hoffman, Alice. *At Risk*. New York: G.P. Putnam's Sons, 1988.

Hoffman, William M. "Dispatches from Aphrodite's War." Review of *Borrowed Time: An AIDS Memoir*, by Paul Monette, and *Mortal Embrace: Living with AIDS*, by Emmanuel Dreuilhe. *New York Times Book Review* 11 Sept. 1988: 3.

James, Caryn. "*At Risk* Author Discusses Fears about AIDS." *New York Times* 18 July 1988: C15.

Lehmann-Haupt, Christopher. "A Family Confronts the AIDS Crisis." Review of *At Risk*, by Alice Hoffman. *New York Times* 4 July 1988: 17.

Mars-Jones, Adam. "Slim." In *The Darker Proof: Stories from a Crisis*, by Edmund White and Adam Mars-Jones. New York: New American Library/Plume, 1988.

Monette, Paul. *Borrowed Time: An AIDS Memoir*. New York: Harcourt Brace Jovanovich, 1988.

———. *Love Alone: Eighteen Elegies for Rog*. New York: St. Martin's Press, 1988.

Peabody, Barbara. *The Screaming Room: A Mother's Journal of Her Son's Struggle with AIDS—A True Story of Love, Dedication, and Courage*. New York: Avon Books, 1987.

Pearson, Carol Lynn. *Good-bye, I Love You*. New York: Random House, 1986.

Rasky, Susan F. "How the Politics Shifted on AIDS Funds." *New York Times* 20 May 1990: 22.

Rieder, Inis, and Patricia Ruppelt, eds. *AIDS: The Women*. San Francisco: Cleis, 1988.

Shepard, Jim. "She Would Have Been Beautiful." Review of *At Risk*, by Alice Hoffman. *New York Times Book Review* 17 July 1988: 7.

Shilts, Randy. *And the Band Played On: Politics, People, and the AIDS Epidemic*. New York: St. Martin's Press, 1987.

Sontag, Susan. "The Way We Live Now." *New Yorker* 24 Nov. 1986: 42–51.

Whitmore, George. *Someone Was Here: Profiles in the AIDS Epidemic*. New York: New American Library, 1988.

Annotated Bibliography

The criteria for inclusion in this bibliography are that the work treats AIDS extensively enough and with enough sympathy and seriousness to make it helpful in combating mistruths about the disease and creating more compassion for those affected by it. The bibliography contains information about a multiplicity of forms beyond traditional literature to give readers a sense of how extensive the artistic response has been to AIDS.

Novels for Adults

Barrus, Tim. *Genocide: The Anthology.* Stamford, Conn.: Knights Press, 1989. A gruesome dystopian collection of apocalyptic prose pieces and poems from a nightmare futuristic society. Although AIDS is not mentioned, its presence is unmistakable as motivating gruesome acts against homosexuals.

Black, Jeff. *Gardy and Erin.* Stamford, Conn.: Knights Press, 1989. Realistic fiction depicting how a man deals with his grief after his lover dies of AIDS.

Bram, Christopher. *In Memory of Angel Clare.* New York: Donald I. Fine, 1989. One of the growing number of memorial tributes, this begins with the AIDS death of a young man's lover and recounts how he deals with his grief and his circle of friends.

Bryan, Jed A. *A Cry in the Desert.* Austin, Tex.: Edward-William Publishing Co., 1987. A dystopian account that imagines deliberate genocide of gay men in Nevada in the early 1980s by Project ERAD.

Bryant, Dorothy. *A Day in San Francisco.* Berkeley, Calif.: Ata Books, 1983. The first novel to deal with AIDS, strongly disliked by the gay community. A mother becomes dismayed at the illness and promiscuous lifestyle she finds in San Francisco's Castro district.

Buck, Charles H. [Hugh Culik]. *The Master Cure.* New York: Jove Publications, 1989. A futuristic thriller about another virus occurring in 1994.

Curzon, Daniel. *The World Can Break Your Heart.* Stanford, Conn.: Knights Press, 1984. A bildungsroman with only the ending specifically relevant to AIDS. Poor, sensitive Benjamin Vance goes to Hollywood to make his fortune but ends up turning tricks instead. When one of his partners gets AIDS, he learns the true meaning of love and compassion.

Davis, Christopher. *Valley of the Shadow.* New York: St. Martin's Press, 1988. A realistic, first-person narrative about a young, wealthy, gay New Yorker and his ex-lover who both die of AIDS.

Duplechan, Larry. *Tangled Up in Blue*. New York: St. Martin's Press, 1989. Realistic fiction that examines how AIDS affects gay-straight relationships.

Exander, Max [Paul Reed]. *SafeStud*. Boston: Alyson Publications, 1985.

———. *LoveSex*. Boston: Alyson Publications, 1986.

———. *ManSex*. San Francisco: Gay Sunshine Press, 1985. All three are erotic safe-sex fiction for gay men.

Feinberg, David B. *Eighty-sixed*. New York: Viking, 1989. An amusing but harrowing before-and-after account of B.J. Rosenthal in Manhattan.

Ferro, Robert. *Second Son*. New York: Crown Publications, 1988. This fourth novel by an artist who has since died mixes realism with science fiction. Both Mark Valerian and his lover Bill Mackey have Kaposi's sarcoma. When Bill gets PCP, a writer friend tells them of another planet, Sirius, where they could emigrate.

Graham, Clayton R. [Larry Ebmeier]. *Tweeds*. Stamford, Conn.: Knights Press, 1987. A funny bildungsroman about a pudgy, midwestern librarian who grows up on a farm loving his handsome best friend. Years later he finds him again in Chicago after his friend has contracted HIV.

Guibert, Hervé. *To The Friend Who Did Not Save My Life*. Trans. Linda Coverdale. New York: Atheneum, 1991. A journal narrating the effects of AIDS on a circle of French artists and intellectuals and the quest for treatment.

Hansen, Joseph. *Early Graves*. New York: Warner Books, 1987. Several PWAs are killed in this murder mystery. Part of a series about L.A. gay insurance investigator and detective Dave Brandstetter.

Hoffman, Alice. *At Risk*. New York: G. P. Putnam's Sons, 1988. The most widely-advertised AIDS novel, about transfusion AIDS in an 11-year-old, white, middle-class girl, and the prejudice she and her family experience.

Johnson, Toby. *Plague: A Novel About Healing*. Boston: Alyson Publications, 1987. A futuristic dystopia in which homophobes, who are repressed gays, plot to use nuclear weapons against PWAs.

McGehee, Peter. *Boys Like Us*. New York: St. Martin's Press, 1991. An honest, humorous look at how AIDS has become a given of gay life today.

Mains, Geoff. *Gentle Warriors*. Stamford, Conn.: Knights Press, 1989. A dystopia about San Francisco AIDS activists who learn that the CIA is involved in the spread of HIV and also possesses its cure. Mains died of AIDS shortly after completing the manuscript and was not able to do much rewriting.

Martin, Kenneth. *Billy's Brother*. London: Gay Men's Press, 1989. The nameless narrator in this detective fiction goes to San Francisco, where his brother has been murdered, and uncovers a scam practiced on PWAs by a holistic health group. A dark view of human nature, straight and gay, prevails.

Maso, Carole. *The Art Lover*. San Francisco: North Point Press, 1990. A woman writer tries to make sense of a world falling apart. The highly experimental postmodern format includes pictures of photographs, details from famous paintings, a novel she is trying to write, and a nonfiction account of her friend Gary Falk's death from AIDS.

Maupin, Armistead. *Baby Cakes.* New York: Harper and Row, 1984. Comic realism, first published in 1983 in the *San Francisco Chronicle* as part of the popular "Tales of the City" series. One of the series' central characters loses his lover to AIDS.

——. *Sure of You.* New York: Harper and Row, 1989. AIDS pervades Maupin's sixth and final volume in the "Tales of the City" series. This humorous but realistic novel documents the momentous changes the disease has created.

Mayes, Sharon. *Immune.* St. Paul, Minn.: New Rivers Press, 1988. One of the first realistic novels to depict female AIDS, shows how infection changes the life of a sexually liberated woman.

Monette, Paul. *Afterlife.* New York: Crown Publications, 1990. Recounts with compassion and grim humor the lives of three AIDS "widowers" trying to keep going in spite of the tremendous grief, rage, and terror each feels.

——. *Halfway Home.* New York: Crown Publications, 1991. Dramatizes the reconciliation between two Irish Catholic brothers, one of whom has AIDS, and examines the meaning of family. A moving depiction of gay love, much more hopeful in mood than most novels about AIDS.

Musto, Michael. *Manhattan on the Rocks.* New York: Holt, Rinehart and Winston, 1989. A gay *Village Voice* columnist recounts the downtown New York club scene, as a heterosexual journalist and his friends try to deny how much AIDS has altered this world.

Purdy, James. *Garments the Living Wear.* San Francisco: City Lights Books, 1989. Realistic fiction by a well-known gay novelist.

Redon, Joel. *Bloodstream.* Stamford, Conn.: Knights Press, 1989. Peter returns to his childhood home, where he must deal with an alcoholic father, a hostile sister, and a loving mother as well as confront his own impending death.

——. *If Not on Earth, Then in Heaven.* New York: St. Martin's Press, 1991. Historical fiction by an HIV-positive author who depicts the prejudice TB sufferers experienced earlier in this century.

Reed, Paul. *Facing It: A Novel of AIDS.* San Francisco: Gay Sunshine Press, 1984. Realistic fiction involving personal villainy and gay and heterosexual love. Set in Manhattan in the summer of 1981.

Rees, David. *The Wrong Apple.* Stamford, Conn.: Knights Press, 1988. A British college professor, on leave in California, falls in love with a young man and brings him home to England, where both test HIV-positive. The young man deserts him for the professor's best friend—a woman—but the professor finally meets someone who accepts his HIV status.

——. *The Colour of His Hair.* Exeter, U.K.: Third House, 1989. Two male teenagers form a relationship; ten years later, not only has the relationship turned sour, but one of them has AIDS.

Schulman, Sarah. *People in Trouble.* New York: E. P. Dutton, 1990. A love triangle between a woman, her husband, and her female lover, written against the background of the AIDS crisis. Describes a group called Justice, modeled on ACT UP.

Stephens, Jack. *Triangulation.* New York: Crown Publications, 1989. Realistic fiction. A heterosexual Baltimore physician is researching AIDS, which creates many personal problems with his lovers and friends.

Uyemoto, Holly. *Rebel Without a Clue.* New York: Crown Publications, 1989. A realistic dramatization of how a heterosexual teenage boy responds when his best friend, a male model, gets AIDS. This is a witty, depressing picture of Valley culture and contemporary high school mores.

Warmbold, Jean. *June Mail.* Sag Harbor, N.Y.: Permanent Press, 1986. Described by Warmbold as a "political thriller" that speculates on where the HIV virus may have originated.

Weir, John. *The Irreversible Decline of Eddie Socket.* New York: Harper and Row, 1989. A darkly comic novel filled with campy dialogue about Hollywood and Broadway.

Novels for Children and Teenagers

Aiello, Barbara, and Jeffrey Shulman. *Friends For Life: Featuring Amy Wilson.* The Kids on the Block Book Series. Frederick, Md.: Twenty-first Century Books, 1988. An excellent short book for any child old enough to read. When members of a fifth-grade video club learn that their sponsor Natalie has AIDS, their reactions provide ways to teach facts and overcome prejudices and fears. For young children.

Cohen, Miriam. *Laura Leonora's 1st Amendment.* New York: Dutton Child Books, 1990. Junior high students in Queens, New York, panic when they learn that a boy with AIDS is going to attend their school. Laura learns important lessons about courage. For junior high school students.

Girard, Linda Walvoord. *Alex, the Kid with AIDS.* Niles, Ill.: Albert Whitman, 1991. A fourth-grade boy with AIDS makes a new friend and learns that, although he is sick, he still cannot misbehave in school. For young children.

Jordan, MaryKate. *Losing Uncle Tim.* Illustrated by Judith Friedman. Niles, Ill.: Albert Whitman, 1989. When Uncle Tim dies of AIDS, Daniel struggles to understand. For young children.

Kerr, M. E. *Night Kites.* New York: Harper and Row, 1987. A realistic dramatization of how a teenager handles AIDS in the older brother he has always adored. Uses the language and concerns of today's youth—friendship, sex, and rock music. For high school students.

Miklowitz, Gloria D. *Good-bye Tomorrow.* New York: Dell, 1987. A well-researched depiction of a high school student who has transfusion AIDS, and the reactions of his classmates and the community. For both junior and high school students.

de Saint Phalle, Niki. *AIDS: You Can't Catch It Holding Hands.* San Francisco: Lapis Press, 1987. A short epistolary novel with colorful graphics—letters from a mother to her son, giving the latest information about AIDS. For both junior and high school students.

Short Stories, Collections, and Novellas

Davis, Christopher. *The Boys in the Bars.* Stamford, Conn.: Knights Press, 1989. According to Davis, all the stories except "History" were written to reflect how the realities of AIDS have altered the lives of gay men.

Delany, Samuel R. "The Tale of Plagues and Carnivals; or, Some Informal Remarks toward the Modular Calculus, Part Five." Appendix A of *Flight from Nevèrÿon.* New York: Bantam Books, 1985. One of the few works to depict AIDS in persons of color. This science fiction story dramatizes AIDS devastation in the inner city among street people, who are mostly homeless addicts or hustlers, and employs a highly complex literary style.

Feinberg, David B. *Spontaneous Combustion.* New York: Viking, 1991. Loosely connected humorous stories in which B.J. Rosenthal, the central character in the novel *Eighty-sixed,* confronts life now that he is HIV-positive.

Gale, Patrick. "The Road to You." *Freezer Counter.* Exeter, U.K.: Third House, 1989. Realistic fiction. A man writes to his HIV-positive lover that in no circumstances will he desert him.

Hot Living. Ed. John Preston. Boston: Alyson Publications, 1985. A collection of early safe-sex pornography.

Leavitt, David. *A Place I've Never Been.* New York: Viking, 1990. The title story and "Gravity" both depict how AIDS affects personal relationships.

Men on Men: Best New Gay Fiction. Ed. George Stambolian. New York: New American Library, 1986. Stories which deal with AIDS are Sam D'Allesandro's "Nothing Ever Just Disappears," Robert Ferro's "Second Son" (a segment of his 1988 novel), John Fox's "Choice," Andrew Holleran's "Friends at Evening," and Edmund White's "An Oracle."

Men on Men 2: Best New Gay Fiction. Ed. George Stambolian. New York: New American Library, 1988. Stories relevant to AIDS are Tim Barrus's "Life Sucks, or Ernest Hemingway Never Slept Here," Christopher Davis's "The Boys in the Bars" (the title story of his own collection), and David B. Feinberg's "Solidarity."

Men on Men 3: Best Gay New Fiction. Ed. George Stambolian. New York: New American Library, 1990. Stories relevant to AIDS are Paul Monette's "Halfway Home" (a portion from his 1991 novel), Matias Viegener's "Twilight of the Gods," Peter Cashorali's "The Ride Home," Robert Haule's "Blond Dog," Alex Jeffers's "My Face in the Mirror," and Andrew Holleran's "Lights in the Valley."

Mills, Joe. "Long to Go." *Oranges and Lemons.* Exeter, U.K.: Third House, 1987. A young man nursing his dying lover hopes that the death will occur fairly soon, for he is already looking forward to a new life.

Pilcher, Darryl S., ed. *Certain Voices.* Boston: Alyson Publications, 1991. Realistic stories about gay men, some of which deal with AIDS.

Rees, David. *Letters to Dorothy.* Exeter, U.K.: Third House, 1990. Stories and essays. Three of the stories deal with AIDS: "Quercus," "Life in Venice," and "The Little Old Ladies of Sidmouth."

———. "Mendocino in October." *Flux.* Exeter, U.K.: Third House, 1988. A middle-aged man, terminally ill with Kaposi's sarcoma, spends a weekend with his closest woman friend and comes to terms with what has happened.

——. "Prague Spring." *The Freezer Counter.* Exeter, U.K.: Third House, 1989. An internationally famous pianist is so distracted by his lover's recent death from AIDS that he almost plays the wrong concerto at a concert in Prague.

Sontag, Susan. "The Way We Live Now." *The New Yorker* 24 Nov. 1986: 42–51. One of the most highly acclaimed early literary works to deal with AIDS. A witty, unsentimental account about the reactions of twenty-six friends toward a man dying of a disease never named.

Spinrad, Norman. "Journals of the Plague Years." *Full Spectrum.* Ed. Lou Aronica and Shawna McCarthy. New York: Bantam Books, 1988. Award-winning science fiction story.

Verghese, Abraham. "Lilacs." *The New Yorker* 14 Oct. 1991: 53–58. A powerful depiction of a PWA choosing when and how he will die.

White, Edmund, ed. *The Faber Book of Gay Short Fiction.* New York: Faber and Faber, 1991. Andrew Holleran's "Sunday Morning: Key West" and White's "Skinned Alive" deal with AIDS.

White, Edmund, and Adam Mars-Jones. *Darker Proof: Stories from a Crisis.* New York: New American Library, 1988. Includes "Running on Empty," "Palace Days," and "An Oracle" by White; and "Slim" by Mars-Jones.

Poetry

Adkins, Kjoseph. "Untitled." *Catalyst* Summer 1991: 39. About the homeless, "lying cement hard on / lonely city streets / coughing up our life / in great gay cities."

Beauchamp, Steven. "Litany: In Time of AIDS." *Catalyst* Spring 1991: 39. A PWA finds "It's hard, this going back / Into the womb" but urges "Come soon, / Oh death. / Come soon."

Boucheron, Robert. *Epitaphs for the Plague Dead.* New York: Ursus Press, 1985. In traditional verse, a variety of persons speak their own epitaphs, including a child killed in the womb by HIV.

Brother to Brother: New Writings by Black Gay Men. Ed. Essex Hemphill. Boston: Alyson Publications, 1991. Contains many poems dealing with AIDS, including Melvin Dixon's "Aunt Ida Pieces a Quilt," Craig G. Harris's "Hope Against Hope," David Frechette's *"Non, Je Ne Regrette Rien,"* and Essex Hemphill's "When My Brother Fell," a tribute to Joseph Beam, who conceived the idea of the collection but died of AIDS before it was completed.

Farmer, Ruth. "AIDS-related Complex." *Catalyst* Summer 1991: 38. About dead Carla, who "clawed her way out of the pit of smack" only to be infected by her "junkie man."

Gunn, Thom. *The Man With Night Sweats.* New York: Farrar, Straus and Giroux, 1992. Most of the poems directly address AIDS; even those which do not do so directly are touched by its images. One of the most powerful is "Lament."

Howe, Marie. "The Promise." In "After AIDS, Gay Art Aims for a New Reality." By Michael Cunningham. *New York Times* 26 Apr. 1992: H17. An excerpt from Howe's collection of verse about her brother, a gay man who died of AIDS.

Klein, Michael, ed. *Poets for Life: Seventy-six Poets Respond to AIDS.* New York: Crown Publications, 1989. Includes "Heartbeats" by Melvin Dixon, "The Plague" by Marvin Bell, "Turtle, Swan" by Mark Doty, "Elegy for John, My Student Dead of AIDS" by Robert Cording, and "What the Intern Saw" by Phillis Levin.

Lassell, Michael. *Decade Dance.* Boston: Alyson Publications, 1990. These poems document gay life in the 80s before and after AIDS; won Lambda Literary Award for best poetry collection.

———. "How to Watch Your Brother Die." *Gay and Lesbian Poetry in Our Time.* Ed. Carl Morse and Joan Larkin. New York: St. Martin's Press, 1988. Also appears in Klein, ed., *Poets For Life.* Told in the second person, about a man who learns to accept the homosexuality and death of his brother simultaneously.

Lynch, Michael. *These Waves of Dying Friends.* New York: Contact II Publications, 1989. These poems focus on what it was like to be a gay activist, a friend and lover of those dying, and a gay parent who is himself infected.

Monette, Paul. *Love Alone: Eighteen Elegies for Rog.* New York: St. Martin's Press, 1988. Written for Monette's lover who died in October 1986.

Phillips, Suzanne. "january 28th." *PWA Coalition Newsline* March 1990: 31. A poem about David and Randy who "got married today / with a real priest / . . . now david . . . says / i can die in peace."

Schreiber, Ron. *John.* Brooklyn, N.Y.: Hanging Loose Press, 1989. A tribute to John MacDonald, Jr., who died of AIDS on November 5, 1986. The poems describe the path from first diagnosis, through illness, treatment, and hospitalization, to death and its aftermath for the surviving lover.

Autobiography, Memoirs, and Personal Essays

Barbo, Beverly. *The Walking Wounded: A Mother's True Story of Her Son's Homosexuality and His Eventual AIDS-related Death!* Lindsborg, Kans.: Carlsons, 1987. A mother describes her son's youth, his coming "out of the closet," and his AIDS illness and death. Barbo now travels all over the country retelling his story and urging people to accept monogamous gay relationships.

Callen, Michael, ed. *Surviving and Thriving with AIDS: Hints for the Newly Diagnosed.* Vol. 1. New York: PWA Coalition, 1987. One of a steadily growing body of anthologies witnessing individual struggles of gay PWAs.

———. *Surviving and Thriving with AIDS. Collected Wisdom.* Vol. 2. New York: PWA Coalition, 1990. Captures many aspects of what it is like to live with AIDS. Sections included are "People of Color and AIDS"; "AIDS and IV Drug Use"; "Family and Friends"; "Love, Sex, and AIDS"; "Pediatric AIDS"; and "Dealing with Disability, Social Security and Medicaid."

Cox, Elizabeth. *Thanksgiving: An AIDS Journal.* New York: Harper and Row, 1990. Cox uses the journal form to vent the anger and frustration she felt caring for her bisexual husband with AIDS. Because she tries to hide the cause of her husband's illness to protect her son, the journal becomes her best friend.

Dreuilhe, Emmanuel. *Mortal Embrace: Living with AIDS.* Trans. (from French *Corps à Corps*) Linda Coverdale. New York: Hill and Wang, 1988. Personal and philosophical reflections by an Egyptian French translator living in New York about his three-year struggle with AIDS.

Glaser, Elizabeth, and Laura Palmer. *In The Absence of Angels: A Hollywood Family's Courageous Story.* New York: G. P. Putnam's Sons, 1991. The wife of actor Paul Michael Glaser tells how she was infected by a blood transfusion in 1981 when she hemorrhaged after giving birth to a daughter, whose mysterious illness at age four revealed that not only she, but her mother and baby brother all carried HIV.

Holleran, Andrew. *Ground Zero.* New York: William Morrow, 1988. Essays by one of the first to write about literature and AIDS.

Hoyle, Jay. *Mark: How a Boy's Courage in Facing AIDS Inspired a Town and the Town's Compassion Lit Up a Nation.* South Bend, Ind.: Langford/Diamond Communications, 1988. A father's account of his hemophiliac son's sixteen-month struggle and the response of Swansea, Massachusetts. Chapter 3 gives the proceedings of a parents' meeting at Joseph Case Junior High School, which the publisher feels may serve as a model for future debate.

Kramer, Larry. *Reports from the Holocaust: The Making of a Gay Activist.* New York: St. Martin's Press, 1989. A collection of Kramer's political writings, including his highly influential 1983 essay "1,112 and Counting."

Lynch, Michael. "Last Onsets: Teaching with AIDS." *Profession* (1990): 32–36. In this collection of essays on language teaching, published by MLA, Lynch explores what it is like to teach his undergraduates about famous death scenes and dying words in literature when everyone in the class knows he is dying of AIDS.

Monette, Paul. *Borrowed Time: An AIDS Memoir.* New York: Harcourt, Brace, Jovanovich, 1988. A moving account of the year and a half before his lover died of AIDS.

———. *Becoming a Man: Half a Life Story.* New York: Harcourt, Brace, Jovanovich, 1992. Monette describes his youth and gradual awareness that he was gay, his sadness at losing lovers and friends, and his own struggle with AIDS, all in a life-affirming style.

Money, J. W. *To All the Girls I've Loved Before: An AIDS Diary.* Boston: Alyson Publications, 1987. Brief, self-reflective essays written during March 1986 while Money was ill; he died in October 1986.

Peabody, Barbara. *The Screaming Room: A Mother's Journal of Her Son's Struggle with AIDS.* New York: Avon Books, 1986. This story begins in December 1983, when few people had heard about the new disease then disparagingly labelled "gay cancer." Useful for teaching fact and compassion.

Pearson, Carol L. *Good-Bye, I Love You.* New York: Jove Publishers, 1988. A wife details the discovery of her husband's bisexuality and later death from AIDS.

Peavey, Fran. *A Shallow Pool of Time.* San Francisco: Crabgrass Press, 1989. Known in the Bay area as the "Atomic Comic" and for her work in grassroots politics, Peavey writes about how having transfusion AIDS politicized her.

Petrow, Steven. *Dancing against the Darkness: A Journey through America in the Age of AIDS.* Lexington, Mass.: Lexington Books, 1990. Profiles of people with AIDS, their families, and friends.

Preston, John, ed. *Personal Dispatches: Writers Confront AIDS.* New York: St. Martin's Press, 1989. Gay and lesbian writers Arnie Kantrowitz, Allan Troxler, Laurence Tate, E. J. Graff, Stephen M. Chapot, Robert Gluck, Andrew Holleran, Steve Beery, Craig Rowland, Stephen Greco, Scott Tucker, Michael Bronski, Edmund White, Robert Dawidoff, and Marea Murray recount their responses and those of others to AIDS.

Reed, Paul. *Serenity: Challenging the Fear of AIDS—From Despair to Hope.* 2d. ed. Berkeley, Calif.: Celestial Arts, 1990. Inspirational essays, chronicling one person's fear of AIDS.

———. *The Q Journal: A Treatment Diary.* San Francisco: Ten Speed Press, 1991. Records Reed's trial of the banned Compound Q.

Rees, David. *Letters to Dorothy.* Exeter, U.K.: Third House, 1990. Stories, essays, and poems, the majority of which are about AIDS or HIV, including an autobiographical essay called "How It Is" about how Rees does and doesn't cope with his HIV problems.

———. *Dog Days, White Nights.* Exeter, U.K.: Third House, 1991. Essays in this collection that deal with AIDS are "Keeping Fit," "Father and Sons," and "Mozart's 'Don Giovanni' as an AIDS Metaphor."

Rieder, Ines, and Patricia Ruppelt, eds. *AIDS: the Women.* Pittsburgh: Cleis Press, 1988. Contains many first-person accounts by women from around the world in their roles as caregivers, HIV-positive or PWAs, prostitutes, health care professionals, lesbians, and educators. Many selections are part of the growing body of "witness" literature.

Ruskin, Cindy. *The Quilt: Stories from the NAMES Project.* New York: Pocket Books, 1988. Includes full-color illustrations of the AIDS memorial quilt, with a narrative text.

Shands, Nancy. *AIDS: The Lonely Voyage.* San Carlos, Calif.: Wide World Publishing, 1988. A compilation of firsthand accounts of what it is like to have AIDS.

White, Ryan, with Ann Marie Cunningham. *Ryan White: My Own Story.* New York: Dial Books, 1991. A personal account by the highly publicized teenager who later died of AIDS.

Whitmore, George. *Someone Was Here: Profiles in the AIDS Epidemic.* New York: St. Martin's Press, 1988. A journalistic account, the final section of which describes the HIV patients at Lincoln Hospital in the South Bronx, most of whom are poor black or Hispanic IV drug users.

Collections of Critical and Analytic Essays, and Individual Articles

Cady, Joseph. "AIDS on the National Stage." *Medical Humanities Review* 6.1 (January 1992): 20–26. This article summarizes the plays written about AIDS through 1991.

Carter, Erica, and Douglas Crimp, eds. *Taking Liberties: AIDS and Cultural Politics.* London: Serpent's Tail, 1989. Essays that look at issues in politics, feminism, medical treatment, eros, and the third world.

Chambers, Lori. "Words = Life." *Rutgers Magazine* Summer 1992: 12–15. Through poetry, professor Rachel Hadas helps men with AIDS find a new voice.

City Lights Review 2 (1988). This issue of the San Francisco literary journal contains a forum on "AIDS, Cultural Life, and the Arts," with poetry, short fiction, essays, and visual art about AIDS by various contributors.

Crimp, Douglas, ed. *AIDS: Cultural Analysis, Cultural Activism.* Cambridge, Mass.: MIT Press, 1987. A collection of now classic critical essays that look at the language, representations, and politics of AIDS, including essays by Crimp, Paula Treichler, Leo Bersani, and Sander L. Gilman.

Miller, James, ed. *Fluid Exchanges: Artists and Critics in the AIDS Crisis.* Toronto: University of Toronto Press, 1992. A collection of essays that evaluate and analyze AIDS images and language in the first decade of the epidemic.

Murphy, Timothy F., and Suzanne Poirier, eds. *Writing AIDS: Gay Literature, Language, and Analysis.* New York: Columbia University Press, 1993. A collection of essays that consider the moral foundations of AIDS representations in AIDS activism, novels, short stories, poetry, and obituaries.

Nelson, Emmanuel S., ed. *AIDS: The Literary Response.* Boston: Twayne, 1992. Essays that look at plague literature and AIDS representations in the United States and other countries.

Stevenson, Sheryl. "Learning through AIDS Poetry." *Feminist Teacher* 5.3 (Spring 1991): 30–33. Stevenson argues that using poetry about AIDS in the classroom can overcome negative attitudes.

Published Plays

Durang, Christopher. *Laughing Wild.* New York: Grove Weidenfeld, 1988. "Seeking Wild," a portion of the play, is included in Osborn, *The Way We Live Now.* One of the characters in this three-part play tries unsuccessfully to practice New Age optimism. At one point he imitates a fundamentalist God, punishing gays with AIDS, indifferent that hemophiliacs, Haitians, and unborn babies will get sick too.

Fierstein, Harvey. *Safe Sex.* New York: Atheneum, 1987. Three one-act plays: "Manny and Jake," "Safe Sex," and "On Tidy Endings." "Safe Sex," reprinted in Osborn, *The Way We Live Now,* begins in the dark, with Ghee and Mead sounding as though they are making love. When the lights go on, however, they are balancing on a see-saw, arguing about how much AIDS has damaged their five-and-a-half-year relationship.

Greenspan, David. *Jack.* In Osborn, *The Way We Live Now.* Strongly influenced by Beckett, Greenspan describes in alternating multivoiced clichés and run-on monologues details of PWA Jack, whose mother beat him, whose bisexual lover went back to his wife, and who eventually died of AIDS.

Hoffman, William M. *As Is.* New York: Random House, 1985. According to Thomas Ryan, "Less political and more personal than *The Normal Heart,* focusing on the renewed love two men experience when one of them is diagnosed with AIDS" (*Spin* Dec. 1988: 86). A revised version appears in Osborn, *The Way We Live Now.*

Kondoleon, Harry. *Zero Positive.* In Osborn, *The Way We Live Now.* In post-AIDS gay New York, everyone is eccentric and unhappy.

Kramer, Larry. *The Normal Heart.* New York: New American Library, 1985. Reprinted in Osborn, *The Way We Live Now.* Based on Kramer's involvement in the formation of the Gay Men's Health Crisis in 1981 and his angry departure in 1983. A powerful work that demands increased government funding and political action.

Kushner, Tony. *Angels in America* (1989). An epic in two parts with many scenes. A portion excerpted in Osborn, *The Way We Live Now,* dramatizes Roy Cohn threatening to ruin his doctor if he reveals Cohn is gay and has AIDS. Other scenes not excerpted sympathetically explore the lives of a drag queen, a straight woman, and a wide range of gay characters.

McNally, Terence. *Andre's Mother.* In Osborn, *The Way We Live Now.* Presented as a teleplay on PBS in 1990. A mother cannot accept her dead son's gayness and blames his lover for his death from AIDS.

Osborn, M. Elizabeth, ed. *The Way We Live Now: American Plays & The AIDS Crisis.* New York: Theatre Communications Group, 1990. An anthology of plays, some published here for the first time, others previously published.

Patrick, Robert. *Pouf Positive.* In *Untold Decades: Seven Comedies of Gay Romance.* Ed. Robert Patrick. New York: St. Martin's Press, 1989. Written for a dead ex-lover who left a message on Patrick's answering machine asking him to "write a comedy about this absurd mess."

Sontag, Susan, and Edward Parone. *The Way We Live Now.* In Osborn, *The Way We Live Now.* Parone adapts Sontag's 1986 *New Yorker* short story in which twenty-six friends respond to the never-named disease of their dying friend.

Vogel, Paula. *The Baltimore Waltz.* An excerpt in Osborn, *The Way We Live Now,* contrasts the fantasy of Anna and her PWA brother Carl that they are traveling in a romantic Europe with slides showing scenes of Johns Hopkins Hospital and surrounding Baltimore where they really are.

Wilson, Lanford. *A Poster of the Cosmos.* In Osborn, *The Way We Live Now.* A one-act play in which a 36-year-old baker memorializes his three-year relationship with hyperactive PWA Johnny.

Unpublished Plays

AIDS Alive (1988). New York's People with AIDS Theater Workshop, whose actors all have AIDS or ARC, founded in 1987. A set of vignettes on performers' experiences with AIDS.

AIDS/US (1986) and *AIDS/US II* (1990). Produced by Artists Confronting AIDS, directed by Michael Kearns, script by James Carroll Pickett based on group interviews. Casts comprise either PWAs or their caregivers. Performed at various sites in the Los Angeles area.

The AIDS Show (1986). Theatre Rhinoceros, San Francisco. A series of sketches, many comic; some performers have AIDS. Some skits appear on a video by Direct Cinema, Ltd.

Alive with AIDS: A Musical Exploration, March 1–26, 1989. Performed at Club Cabaret at the Club Cafe, Boston. PWAs, their friends and relatives, and health care workers join artists in a production which mixes comedy with pathos.

Bowne, Alan. *Beirut* (1987). Performed at New York's Westside Arts Theater, starring Michael David Morrison and Laura San Giacomo. The first play to depict AIDS in heterosexuals. The futuristic work is based on *Romeo and Juliet.*

Branner, Bernard Djola, Brian Freeman, and Eric Gupton. *PoMo Afro Homos* (Post-Modern African-American Homosexuals). A San Francisco–based trio who perform trenchant tragicomic sketches about black gay life.

Bumbalo, Victor. *Adam and the Experts* (1989). Produced by New York's gay community company Three Dollar Bill Theater. Dramatizes the illness and death of Bumbalo's friend, the journalist George Whitmore.

Chapman, James. *Our Young Black Men are Dying and Nobody Seems to Care* (1990). Performed by Living the Dream in New York's Castillo Cultural Center, Boston's Strand Theatre, and also in Dayton, Ohio. Chapman uses music, poetry, and humor to tell the stories of several men threatened by a variety of ills: poverty, homelessness, gang violence, drugs, and AIDS.

Chesley, Robert. *Night Sweat* (1984). The first play about AIDS.

———. *Jerker; or, the Helping Hand* (1986). A one-act play in which two strangers conduct their entire relationship over the phone.

Clarke, Bruce. *The Inner Web* (1990). An autobiographical account of Clark's experiences with AIDS. He wrote the play as therapy and directed and starred in it at Boston's Clarendon Street Theater.

Copi. *Grand Finale* (1987). A French black comedy about an actor dying of AIDS. Translated by Michael Feingold and premiered in New York in 1991.

Edelstein, Lisa. *Positive Me* (1989). Performed at New York's La Mama. A musical intended to educate teenagers about AIDS.

Elovich, Richard. *If Men Could Talk, the Stories They Could Tell* (1990). A one-man piece which focuses on a gay man's struggle with AIDS.

Finn, William, and James Lapine. *Falsettoland* (1991). Music and lyrics by Finn, directed by Graciela Daniele. A musical, the third in a trilogy chronicling the life of Marvin, a young, compulsive Jewish man, who, in this play, learns he has AIDS.

Gurney, A. R. *The Old Boy* (1991). Performed by New York's Playwrights Horizons. Flashbacks and recollections by friends tell of a middle-aged WASP who came out of the closet and committed suicide after contracting HIV.

Holsclaw, Doug. *The Life of the Party* (1987). A romantic comedy in which four healthy gay men discuss safe sex, developed from the 1986 *AIDS Show.*

Kramer, Larry. *The Destiny of Me* (1992). A play filled with sorrow and rage; yet at one point, a fiercely angry, middle-aged man with AIDS unites with his unhappy, rebellious, adolescent self to sing a song of love and hope from *South Pacific.*

———. *Just Say No* (1988). A satire of federal policy about AIDS.

———. *Reports from the Holocaust: The Making of an AIDS Activist* (1990). The Manbites Dog Theater Company of Durham, North Carolina, adapted the title essay from Kramer's collection into a one-act play, which they performed at New York's Public Theater.

Lipsky, Jon. *Dreaming with an AIDS Patient* (1989). Written and directed by Lipsky. Adapted from Robert Bosnak's nonfiction account of the interaction between a gay patient and his psychiatrist, both characters played by the same actor. Essentially a monologue, the play merges the real with the surreal.

Lucas, Craig. *Prelude to a Kiss.* Written by the author of AIDS film *Longtime Companion,* the play never mentions AIDS, nor are the characters in any high-risk groups, but the play can be viewed as an AIDS allegory. Released in 1992 as a major motion picture.

MacLean, David. *Quarantine of the Mind* (1990). A solo work exploring gay sexuality in the time of AIDS, produced by Boston's Mobius Theatre Company.

McNally, Terrence. *Lips Together, Teeth Apart* (1991). Premiered in June 1991 at the Manhattan Theater Club; had long run at New York's Lucille Lortel Theater; directed by John Tilinger. Two couples spend the fourth of July on Fire Island, where they struggle to deal with homophobia and their fear of AIDS.

Mellon, James J. *An Unfinished Song* (1992). Book, music, and lyrics by Mellon; directed by Michael Rafkin; produced by TriAngle Productions and Mad Horse Theater Company of Portland, Maine. A musical about four friends who gather after the funeral of a gay composer, using flashbacks to depict his life.

People with AIDS Theatre Workshop (1988). Founded in 1988 by Sylvia Stein and Nick Pippin. A group of PWAs performed at New York's Don't Tell Mama cabaret "stories ranging from bittersweet to angry to exceptionally funny" (Thomas S. Ryan, *Spin* Dec. 1988: 86).

Russell, Bill. *Elegies for Angels, Punks and Raging Queens (an AIDS Anthology)* (1990). Written and staged by Russel, inspired by his first viewing of the NAMES quilt and by Edgar Lee Master's *Spoon River Anthology.* Thirty poems are read by thirty actors who are accompanied by blues, jazz, and gospel music.

Sheppard, David. *Heartstrings* (1986). Initially inspired by Etty Hillesum's Auschwitz diary *An Interrupted Life.* Quotes from a diary connected by an allegory of an American small town enveloped in a cloud where lack of sunlight is creating a wasting disease. Uses original arrangements of songs by Simon and Garfunkel, Irving Berlin and others. Performed around the country in 1989 and 1990 at various AIDS benefits.

Spencer, Stuart. *Last Outpost at the End of the World* (1987). This part of the Ensemble Studio Theater's one-act marathon dramatizes how people have been affected by AIDS.

Swados, Robin. *A Quiet End* (1990). Premiered in New York. Three gay men share their experiences in an AIDS hospice.

van Italie, Jean-Claude. *Ancient Boys* (1991). This play uses flashbacks and the words of friends to tell about a sculptor who died of AIDS.

West, Cheryl. *Before It Hits Home* (1991). Performed at New York's Public Theater. A dramatization of how an African-American family reacts when the eldest son, a bisexual musician, gets AIDS.

Television Dramas, Independent Films, and Videos

"Broadcasters Respond to AIDS," a complete listing of videos and radio programs made up to 1989, was published by KIDSNET/AIDS, 6856 Eastern Avenue, NW, Suite 208, Washington, DC 20012.

Adair, Peter. *Absolutely Positive.* Presented June 18, 1991, on PBS's "P.O.V." series. Based on interviews with eleven different HIV-positive people. A deeply affecting work by a filmmaker who is himself HIV-positive.

The AIDS Show. Direct Cinema Ltd. (1986). A series of skits performed by the San Francisco Theatre Rhinoceros, interspersed with interviews and voiceovers about the emotional effects of the disease.

AIDS–Wise, No Lies. New Day; written and directed by David Current and Anne Rutledge. Ten young people whose lives are affected by AIDS reveal thoughts, feelings, and experiences in their own words from their own environments.

All of Us and AIDS. Written and directed by Peer Education Health Resources and Catherine Jordan. Nine teenagers make a videotape on postponing sexual intercourse, condom buying and use, personal fears of AIDS exposure, gay sexual decisions, and conflicting attitudes.

Are You With Me? AIDSfilms (1989); directed by Neema Barnet; screenplay by Marian Warrington. An African-American mother and daughter discuss the need for safe sex. Distributed by Select Media.

An Early Frost. NBC (1985); written by Ron Cowen and Daniel Lipman; starring Ben Gazzara and Aidan Quinn. A gay lawyer from Chicago has AIDS and tries to regain the love of his disapproving father.

Epstein, Robert, and Jeffrey Friedman. *Common Threads: Stories from the Quilt.* HBO (1989). This Oscar-winning documentary tells the stories behind five of those memorialized in the NAMES Quilt.

Huff, Bob. *Rockville Is Burning* (1988). AIDS activists take over a television station and begin broadcasting a radically different version of the epidemic.

Hutt, Robyn, Sandra Elgear, and David Meieran. *Voices from the Front* (1992). Produced by New York's Testing the Limits Collective. Persons with AIDS and AIDS activists tell their stories and explain their strategies for gaining greater control over health care, research, and funding.

In a New Light. ABC (July 11, 1992). Two-hour special/musical tribute about AIDS, based largely on *Heartstrings,* the 1986 musical, written by David Sheppard, initially inspired by Etty Hillesum's Auschwitz diary *An Interrupted Life.*

In the Shadow of Love. Coproduced by PBS and ABC, September 18–19, 1991; written by Gordon Rayfield; directed by Consuelo Gonzalez; starring Jennifer

Dundas, Lisa Vidal, and Harvey Fierstein. A frank presentation of teenage sex and facts about risky behavior.

Intimate Contact. HBO (1987); starring Claire Bloom and Raymond Massey. A wife who learns her husband has contracted AIDS from a prostitute on a business trip comes to terms with the dilemma as her anger gradually gives way to a determination to play a public role in fighting the disease.

A Letter from Brian. American Red Cross Production (1987). A twenty-minute film for high school students. Tells of a seventeen-year-old girl who receives a letter from an old boyfriend who has contracted AIDS; she decides she will not become sexually involved with a new boyfriend.

Longtime Companion. Goldwyn (1990). Directed by Norman Rene; screenplay by Craig Lucas; starring Stephen Cassidy, Patrick Cassidy, Bruce Davison, Mary-Louise Parker, and Campbell Scott. The only major commercial film to focus totally on AIDS traces the course of the epidemic on a loosely-knit group of New York gay men and friends over a nine-year period.

Ojos Que No Ven [Eyes That Fail to See] (1987). Produced for the Latino AIDS project using the popular *telenovela* (a kind of soap opera) format, addressed specifically to Chicanos in the San Francisco Bay area. Practical information about safe sex, clean needles, and AIDS testing woven into drama.

Our Sons. ABC (1991). Starring Julie Andrews and Ann-Margaret. Two mothers of gay sons, one accepting, one rejecting.

The Ryan White Story. ABC (1989); Alan Landsburg Production Co.; starring Judith Light and Lukas Haas. A white, hemophiliac boy is ostracized by schoolmates and neighbors because he has AIDS.

Seriously Fresh. AIDSfilms (1989); directed by Reggie Life; screenplay by Jamal Joseph. Focuses on the lives of four young African-American men and their older friend who becomes ill with HIV. Uses humor to address many crucial issues.

Sherwood, Bill. *Parting Glances* (1986). A moving drama that interweaves a subplot about a PWA into the main story.

Smith, Mona. *Her Giveaway.* Women Make Movies (1988). Carole Lafavor, a member of the Ojibwa tribe, activist, mother, and registered nurse, is a PWA. Lafavor relates how she has come to terms with AIDS by combining her traditional beliefs and healing practices with western medicine.

Spiro, Ellen. *DiAna's Hair Ego: AIDS Info Upfront* (1990). A half-hour account of a Columbia, South Carolina, hairdresser who began by distributing free, gift-wrapped condoms to her customers and later founded the South Carolina AIDS Education Network.

Tongues Untied. Presented on PBS's "Point of View" series, July 16, 1991; directed by Marlon Riggs. One of the few works to explore the gay black experience, this fifty-five-minute film employs a number of different artistic media, including poetry, song, dance, rap, and clips from Eddie Murphy's standup routine and a scene from Spike Lee's *School Daze,* both of which show the strong homophobia felt by many blacks.

Vida. AIDSfilms (1989). Directed by Lourdes Porpillo, screenplay by Anna

Marie Simo. A story about condom use among teenagers. Available in English and Spanish from Select Media.

Video against AIDS (1990). Curated by John Greyson and Bill Horrigan, produced by Kat Horsfield. Three programs, two hours long each, covering three AIDS-connected themes. Available from Video Data Bank in Chicago and New York and V Tape in Toronto.

Voices from the Front. Testing the Limits Collective (1990). A political documentary depicting the problems PWAs face in finding treatment and housing, as well as the issues that confront AIDS activists in trying to educate the public.

Mixed Media, Miscellaneous

Crimp, Douglas, with Adam Rolston. *AIDS Demo Graphics.* Seattle: Bay State, 1990. Graphics used by New York's ACT UP, plus a history of the group's origin and activities.

Eggan, Ferd. *Your LIFE Story by Someone Else.* Chicago: Editorial Coqui, 1989. Explodes with anger, as Eggan puts together poems and stories collaborated on by a group of Chicago graphic artists.

Howard, Billy. *Epitaphs for the Living: Words and Images in the Time of AIDS.* Introduction by Lonnie D. Kleiver. Dallas: Southern Methodist University Press, 1989. PWAs write their own epitaphs, with photographs by Howard.

A hundred LEGENDS. New York: Design Industries Foundation for AIDS, 1990. A portfolio of art, poetry, prose, and music by over 100 men, women and children with AIDS. Reproductions of the artists' work, along with an audio cassette of music.

Piersma, Lyman, ed. *Going to Camp: A Meditation about AIDS, Quarantine, Exile and Personal Loss.* Rosendale, N.Y.: Women's Studio Workshop, 1990. A folio of visual and textual images designed and executed by Lyman Piersma. Twenty contributors provided color photocopies, silkscreens, rubber stamps, photography, poetry, and fiction. Limited edition of 65.

Robbins, Trina, Bill Sienkiewicz, and Robert Triptow, eds. *Strip AIDS USA.* San Francisco: Last Gasp, 1988. Collection of cartoons about AIDS.

Music

RAP

Fat Boys "Protect Yourself." *Crushin'.* Tin Pan Apple Records, 1987.

CLASSICAL

Adams, John. "The Wound Dresser." Based on a poem by Walt Whitman about his nursing experiences in Civil War; Adams, composer of the opera *Nixon in China,* applies the poem to today's AIDS patients.

Corigliano, John. Symphony No. 1. "The first major musical AIDS memorial," according to Richard Dyer (*Boston Globe* 12 July 1991: 51). 1992 Grammy winner.

Notes on Contributors

Laurel Brodsley, R.N., Ph.D., M.P.H., is a lecturer in the UCLA English department. She has worked at Girton College, Cambridge, held a Pew Fellowship at the UCLA/Rand Center for Health Policy, and done clinical nursing.

Jed A. Bryan is a native of Utah who now lives on California's central coast. He taught for ten years before becoming a designer of computer information systems for education. Besides *A Cry in the Desert* (1987), he has written *Sacred Cows* (1989).

Joseph Cady teaches literature and medicine in the Division of Medical Humanities at the University of Rochester Medical School, and gay and lesbian literature at the New School for Social Research. He has also taught at Columbia and Rutgers and was a practicing psychotherapist in New York. His essays and poems have appeared in *American Studies, Socialist Review, Radical Teacher, American Poetry Review, Massachusetts Review,* and elsewhere.

Sam Coale has taught American literature at Wheaton College, Massachusetts, since 1968. He is the author of *In Hawthorne's Shadow: American Romance from Melville to Mailer* (1985), *William Styron Revisited* (1991), and works on John Cheever, Anthony Burgess, and Paul Theroux. A recipient of Fulbright awards and a National Endowment for the Humanities grant, he has taught and traveled extensively in Eastern Europe, the Middle East, and South America.

Michael Denneny, author of *Lovers: The Story of Two Men* (1979) and *Decent Passions: Real Stories about Love* (1983) is a senior editor at St. Martin's Press and the general editor of their Stonewall Inn Editions.

Melvin Dixon, author of *Trouble the Water* (1989), *Red Leaves* (1990), *Vanishing Rooms* (1991), and a volume of poetry, *Change of Territory* (1983) died of AIDS in 1992. He has received fellowships in poetry and fiction from the National Endowment for the Arts and the New York Arts Foundation. His work has appeared in many journals and anthologies, including *In the Life* (1986), *Men on Men 2: Best New Gay Fiction* (1988), *Poets for Life: 76 Poets Respond to AIDS* (1989), and *Brother to Brother* (1991).

Larry Ebmeier, who frequently writes under the name Clayton R. Graham, is the author of *A Man of Taste* (1984), *Walkin' Matilda* (1984), *Tweeds* (1987), and *Engineman* (1992). A graduate of the University of Nebraska's College of Pharmacy, he currently is a hospital pharmacist in Lincoln, Nebraska.

DAVID B. FEINBERG is the author of the novel *Eighty-sixed* (1989) and the short story collection *Spontaneous Combustion* (1991). Originally from Lynn, Massachusetts, he lives now in New York City. He received a B.S. in mathematics from MIT and an M.A. in linguistics from NYU. He joined ACT UP/NY shortly after testing HIV-positive.

WILLIAM GREENWAY has published two books of poetry: *Pressure under Grace* (1982) and *Where We've Been* (1987). He is an associate professor of English at Youngstown State University.

JAMES W. JONES, associate professor of German at Central Michigan University, received his Ph.D. from the University of Wisconsin. He has written on AIDS discourses as well as on German gay literature. His study *"We of the Third Sex": Literary Representations of Homosexuality in Wilhelmine Germany* was published in 1990.

M. E. KERR is the author of thirteen novels for young adults and the autobiographical *Me, Me, Me, Me, Me: Not a Novel* (1983). Born Marijane Meaker, she attended the University of Missouri and worked in publishing in New York City for twenty years before the appearance of her first M. E. Kerr novel, *Dinky Hocker Shoots Smack!* (1972), which was adapted into an ABC–TV "Afterschool Special." She has also written adult mysteries as Vin Packer and other adult books as M. J. Meaker.

MICHAEL LYNCH, one of Canada's foremost gay rights and AIDS activists, was forty-six when he died in 1991. Author of the poetry collection *These Waves of Dying Friends* (1989), associate professor of literature at the University of Toronto since 1971, and a native of North Carolina, he was editor for many years of the *Lesbian and Gay Studies Newsletter* and helped found AIDS Action Now, a group devoted exclusively to influencing public policy. Lynch, who is survived by a son, Stefan, founded the group Gay Fathers in 1978.

SHARON MAYES, who received a Ph.D. in sociology from Yale, is the author of *Immune* (1988), a novel about AIDS, as well as numerous short stories and poems. She lives with her husband in California, where she operates an African stone sculpture gallery while working on a new novel, *An Unlikely Terrorist.*

PAUL MONETTE is the author of *Love Alone: 18 Elegies for Rog* (1988) and eleven other works of fiction, poetry, and movie novelizations, including *Borrowed Time: An AIDS Memoir* (1988), *Afterlife* (1989), and *Halfway Home* (1991).

JUDITH LAURENCE PASTORE received her Ph.D. from Harvard and is a professor of English at the University of Massachusetts at Lowell, where she coordinates the Technology, Society, and Values program. Her publications include articles on Samuel Richardson's *Pamela,* Don DeLillo, Alice Hoffman's *At Risk,* and "Using Literature to Understand AIDS."

JOEL REDON was born in Georgia, studied writing with Paul Bowles in Morocco and with Elizabeth Pollet at NYU, and wrote columns and reviews for the *New York Native* in 1986–87. He is the author of *Bloodstream* (1989), *If Not on Earth, Then in Heaven* (1991), and the recently completed *Road to Zena.*

Paul Reed, the San Francisco-based author of *Facing It* (1984), was one of the first to write about the need for safe sex. His other works include *Serenity* (1991), a collection of inspirational essays, and *The O Journal* (1991), as well as three books of safe-sex erotica written under the pseudonym Max Exander.

David Rees lives in Exeter, England, and is the author of *The Wrong Apple* (1988) and *The Colour of His Hair* (1989) as well as collections of short stories, essays, and poetry, including *Flux* (1988), *Letters to Dorothy* (1990), and *Dog Days, White Nights* (1991). His most recent works are an autobiography, *Not for Your Hands* (1992), and *Packing It In* (1992), an account of traveling with AIDS in Europe, North America, and Australasia.

May Sarton, a feminist novelist, poet, and essayist, lives in York, Maine. Among her many works are *The Small Room* (1961), *Joanna and Ulysses* (1963), *Mrs. Stevens Hears the Mermaids Singing* (1965), and *Kinds of Love* (1970).

Eve Kosofsky Sedgwick is a professor of English at Duke University. Her critical works include *Between Men* (1986) and *The Epistemology of the Closet* (1991).

Sandra W. Stephan, an associate professor of English at Youngstown State University, teaches literary AIDS at the Northeast Ohio Universities College of Medicine (NEOUCOM) and conducted sessions on Literary AIDS at the NEH Institute for Humanities and Medicine at Hiram College, Ohio, in 1991–92. She serves on the advisory board of the Center for Literature, Medicine, and the Health Care Professions, a Hiram College/NEOUCOM project.